R0006536015

D0463872

Prediabetes and Diabetes Prevention

Guest Editor

MICHAEL BERGMAN, MD

MEDICAL CLINICS ʼ OF NORTH AMERICA

www.medical.theclinics.com

March 2011 • Volume 95 • Number 2

SAUNDERS an imprint of ELSEVIER, Inc.

W.B. SAUNDERS COMPANY
A Division of Elsevier Inc.

1600 John F. Kennedy Boulevard • Suite 1800 • Philadelphia, Pennsylvania 19103-2899

http://www.theclinics.com

MEDICAL CLINICS OF NORTH AMERICA Volume 95, Number 2
March 2011 ISSN 0025-7125, ISBN-13: 978-1-4557-0467-5

Editor: Rachel Glover
Developmental Editor: Jessica Demetriou

© **2011 Elsevier Inc. All rights reserved.**

This journal and the individual contributions contained in it are protected under copyright by Elsevier, and the following terms and conditions apply to their use:

Photocopying
Single photocopies of single articles may be made for personal use as allowed by national copyright laws. Permission of the Publisher and payment of a fee is required for all other photocopying, including multiple or systematic copying, copying for advertising or promotional purposes, resale, and all forms of document delivery. Special rates are available for educational institutions that wish to make photocopies for non-profit educational classroom use. For information on how to seek permission visit www.elsevier.com/permissions or call: (+44) 1865 843830 (UK)/(+1) 215 239 3804 (USA).

Derivative Works
Subscribers may reproduce tables of contents or prepare lists of articles including abstracts for internal circulation within their institutions. Permission of the Publisher is required for resale or distribution outside the institution. Permission of the Publisher is required for all other derivative works, including compilations and translations (please consult www.elsevier.com/permissions).

Electronic Storage or Usage
Permission of the Publisher is required to store or use electronically any material contained in this journal, including any article or part of an article (please consult www.elsevier.com/permissions). Except as outlined above, no part of this publication may be reproduced, stored in a retrieval system or transmitted in any form or by any means, electronic, mechanical, photocopying, recording or otherwise, without prior written permission of the Publisher.

Notice
No responsibility is assumed by the Publisher for any injury and/or damage to persons or property as a matter of products liability, negligence or otherwise, or from any use or operation of any methods, products, instructions or ideas contained in the material herein. Because of rapid advances in the medical sciences, in particular, independent verification of diagnoses and drug dosages should be made.

Although all advertising material is expected to conform to ethical (medical) standards, inclusion in this publication does not constitute a guarantee or endorsement of the quality or value of such product or of the claims made of it by its manufacturer.

Medical Clinics of North America (ISSN 0025-7125) is published bimonthly by Elsevier Inc., 360 Park Avenue South, New York, NY 10010-1710. Months of issue are January, March, May, July, September, and November. Periodicals postage paid at New York, NY, and additional mailing offices. Subscription prices are USD 218 per year for US individuals, USD 404 per year for US institutions, USD 110 per year for US students, USD 277 per year for Canadian individuals, USD 525 per year for Canadian institutions, USD 173 per year for Canadian students, USD 336 per year for international individuals, USD 525 per year for international institutions and USD 173 per year for international students. To receive student/resident rate, orders must be accompanied by name of affiliated institution, date of term, and the *signature* of program/residency coordinator on institution letterhead. Orders will be billed at individual rate until proof of status is received. Foreign air speed delivery is included in all *Clinics* subscription prices. All prices are subject to change without notice. **POSTMASTER:** Send address changes to *Medical Clinics of North America*, Elsevier Health Sciences Division, Subscription Customer Service, 3251 Riverport Lane, Maryland Heights, MO 63043. **Customer Service: Telephone: 1-800-654-2452** (U.S. and Canada); **1-314-447-8871** (outside U.S. and Canada). **Fax: 1-314-447-8029.** E-mail: **journalscustomerservice-usa@elsevier.com** (for print support); **journalsonlinesupport-usa@elsevier.com** (for online support).

Reprints. For copies of 100 or more of articles in this publication, please contact the Commercial Reprints Department, Elsevier Inc., 360 Park Avenue South, New York, NY 10010-1710. Tel.: 212-633-3812; Fax: 212-462-1935; E-mail: reprints@elsevier.com.

Medical Clinics of North America is also published in Spanish by McGraw-Hill Interamericana Editores S. A., P.O. Box 5-237, 06500 Mexico, D.F., Mexico.

Medical Clinics of North America is covered in *MEDLINE/PubMed (Index Medicus), Current Contents, ASCA, Excerpta Medica, Science Citation Index,* and *ISI/BIOMED.*

Printed in the United States of America.

GOAL STATEMENT

The goal of *Medical Clinics of North America* is to keep practicing physicians up to date with current clinical practice by providing timely articles reviewing the state of the art in patient care.

ACCREDITATION

The *Medical Clinics of North America* is planned and implemented in accordance with the Essential Areas and Policies of the Accreditation Council for Continuing Medical Education (ACCME) through the joint sponsorship of the University of Virginia School of Medicine and Elsevier. The University of Virginia School of Medicine is accredited by the ACCME to provide continuing medical education for physicians.

The University of Virginia School of Medicine designates this educational activity for a maximum of 15 *AMA PRA Category 1 Credits*™ for each issue, 90 credits per year. Physicians should only claim credit commensurate with the extent of their participation in the activity.

The American Medical Association has determined that physicians not licensed in the US who participate in this CME activity are eligible for a maximum of 15 *AMA PRA Category 1 Credits*™ for each issue, 90 credits per year.

Credit can be earned by reading the text material, taking the CME examination online at http://www.theclinics.com/home/cme, and completing the evaluation. After taking the test, you will be required to review any and all incorrect answers. Following completion of the test and evaluation, your credit will be awarded and you may print your certificate.

FACULTY DISCLOSURE/CONFLICT OF INTEREST

The University of Virginia School of Medicine, as an ACCME accredited provider, endorses and strives to comply with the Accreditation Council for Continuing Medical Education (ACCME) Standards of Commercial Support, Commonwealth of Virginia statutes, University of Virginia policies and procedures, and associated federal and private regulations and guidelines on the need for disclosure and monitoring of proprietary and financial interests that may affect the scientific integrity and balance of content delivered in continuing medical education activities under our auspices.

The University of Virginia School of Medicine requires that all CME activities accredited through this institution be developed independently and be scientifically rigorous, balanced and objective in the presentation/discussion of its content, theories and practices.

All authors/editors participating in an accredited CME activity are expected to disclose to the readers relevant financial relationships with commercial entities occurring within the past 12 months (such as grants or research support, employee, consultant, stock holder, member of speakers bureau, etc.). The University of Virginia School of Medicine will employ appropriate mechanisms to resolve potential conflicts of interest to maintain the standards of fair and balanced education to the reader. Questions about specific strategies can be directed to the Office of Continuing Medical Education, University of Virginia School of Medicine, Charlottesville, Virginia.

The faculty and staff of the University of Virginia Office of Continuing Medical Education have no financial affiliations to disclose.

The authors/editors listed below have identified no professional or financial affiliations for themselves or their spouse/partner:
Mehmet Agirbasli, MD; Gerald S. Berenson, MD; Michael Bergman, MD, FACP (Guest Editor); Martin Buysschaert, MD, PhD; Wei Chen, MD, PhD; Stephen Colagiuri, MB BS, FRACP; Jill P. Crandall, MD; Ele Ferrannini, MD; Rachel Glover, (Acquisitions Editor); Patricia Iozzo, MD; Sofiya Milman, MD; Quoc Manh Nguyen, MD, MPH; A. Ramachandran, MD, PhD, DSc, FRCP (London), FRCP (Edinburg); Anpalakan Sathasivam, MD; Peter E.H. Schwarz, MD, PhD; Jonathan Shaw, MD, FRACP, FRCP(UK); C. Snehalatha, MSc, DPhil, DSc; Sathanur R. Srinivasan, PhD; and Andrew Wolf, MD (Test Author).

The authors/editors listed below identified the following professional or financial affiliations for themselves or their spouse/partner:
Amalia Gastaldelli, PhD is an industry funded research/investigator and consultant for F. Hoffmann-La Roche Ltd., and is an industry funded research/investigator for Eli Lilly and Company.
William H. Herman, MD, MPH is a consultant for Amylin/Lilly, Johnson&Johnson, Pfizer, and Sanofi-Aventis.
Robert E. Ratner, MD is an industry funded research/investigator and is on the Advisory Committee/Board for Amylin Pharmaceuticals, NovoNordisk, and Sanofi-Aventis, and is an industry funded research/investigator for GSK.

Disclosure of Discussion of Non-FDA Approved Uses for Pharmaceutical Products and/or Medical Devices.
The University of Virginia School of Medicine, as an ACCME provider, requires that all faculty presenters identify and disclose any off-label uses for pharmaceutical and medical device products. The University of Virginia School of Medicine recommends that each physician fully review all the available data on new products or procedures prior to clinical use.

TO ENROLL

To enroll in the Medical Clinics of North America Continuing Medical Education program, call customer service at 1-800-654-2452 or visit us online at http://www.theclinics.com/home/cme. The CME program is available to subscribers for an additional fee of USD 228.

RELATED INTEREST

Endocrinology and Metabolism Clinics of North America, September 2010
(Volume 39, Issue 3)
Type I Diabetes
Desmond A. Schatz, MD, Michael J. Haller, MD, and Mark A. Atkinson, PhD,
Guest Editors

VISIT US ONLINE!
Access your subscription at:
www.theclinics.com

Contributors

GUEST EDITOR

MICHAEL BERGMAN, MD, FACP
Clinical Professor of Medicine, Department of Medicine, Division of Endocrinology, New York University School of Medicine, New York, New York

AUTHORS

MEHMET AGIRBASLI, MD
Department of Cardiology, Marmara University, Istanbul, Turkey

GERALD S. BERENSON, MD
Tulane Center for Cardiovascular Health, Tulane University Health Sciences Center, New Orleans, Louisiana

MICHAEL BERGMAN, MD, FACP
Clinical Professor of Medicine, Department of Medicine, Division of Endocrinology, New York University School of Medicine, New York, New York

MARTIN BUYSSCHAERT, MD, PhD
Professor of Medicine and Chief, Department of Endocrinology and Diabetology, University Clinic Saint-Luc, Université Catholique de Louvain (UCL), Brussels, Belgium

WEI CHEN, MD, PhD
Tulane Center for Cardiovascular Health, Tulane University Health Sciences Center, New Orleans, Louisiana

STEPHEN COLAGIURI, MB BS, FRACP
Professor of Metabolic Health, Boden Institute of Obesity, Nutrition and Exercise, University of Sydney, Sydney, New South Wales, Australia

JILL P. CRANDALL, MD
Professor of Clinical Medicine and Director of Diabetes Clinical Trials Unit, Diabetes Research and Training Center; Division of Endocrinology, Albert Einstein College of Medicine, Bronx, New York

ELE FERRANNINI, MD
Professor of Medicine, Department of Internal Medicine, University of Pisa School of Medicine, Pisa, Italy

AMALIA GASTALDELLI, PhD
Senior Investigator, CNR Institute of Clinical Physiology, Pisa, Italy

WILLIAM H. HERMAN, MD, MPH
Stefan S. Fajans/GlaxoSmithKline Professor of Diabetes, Professor of Internal Medicine and Epidemiology, Division of Metabolism, Endocrinology and Diabetes, University of Michigan, Ann Arbor, Michigan

PATRICIA IOZZO, MD
Senior Investigator, CNR Institute of Clinical Physiology, Pisa, Italy

SOFIYA MILMAN, MD
Fellow in Endocrinology, Division of Endocrinology, Montefiore Medical Center, Albert Einstein College of Medicine, Bronx, New York

QUOC MANH NGUYEN, MD, MPH
Tulane Center for Cardiovascular Health, Tulane University Health Sciences Center, New Orleans, Louisiana

A. RAMACHANDRAN, MD, PhD, DSc, FRCP (London), FRCP (Edinburg)
President, India Diabetes Research Foundation; Chairman and Managing Director, Dr A. Ramachandran's Diabetes Hospitals, Egmore, Chennai, Tamil Nadu, India

ROBERT E. RATNER, MD
Senior Scientist, MedStar Health Research Institute, Hyattsville, Maryland; Professor of Medicine, Division of Endocrinology, Georgetown University School of Medicine, Washington, DC

ANPALAKAN SATHASIVAM, MD
Fellow in Endocrinology and Metabolism, Division of Endocrinology, Georgetown University School of Medicine, Washington, DC

PETER E.H. SCHWARZ, MD, PhD
Department for Prevention and Care of Diabetes, Medical Clinic III, University Clinic Carl Gustav Carus at the Technical University Dresden, Dresden, Germany

JONATHAN SHAW, MD, FRACP, FRCP(UK)
Associate Professor, Baker IDI Heart and Diabetes Institute, Melbourne, Australia

C. SNEHALATHA, MSc, DPhil, DSc
Director of Research, India Diabetes Research Foundation; Head, Department of Biochemistry, Dr A. Ramachandran's Diabetes Hospitals, Egmore, Chennai, Tamil Nadu, India

SATHANUR R. SRINIVASAN, PhD
Tulane Center for Cardiovascular Health, Tulane University Health Sciences Center, New Orleans, Louisiana

Contents

Diabetes evolves through prediabetes, defined as impaired fasting glucose (IFG) and/or impaired glucose tolerance (IGT). Subjects with IFG/IGT have an increased risk of developing diabetes and a higher prevalence of cardio-vascular disease than normoglycemic individuals. However, there is considerable evidence that glucose levels lower than those meeting the current definition of prediabetes may also be associated with similar concerns, particularly in high-risk individuals in accordance with a continuous glycemic risk perspective. Therefore, an absolute definition of prediabetes may underestimate the implications and vastness of this disorder. Research should focus on these aspects to minimize the risk of developing a preventable condition.

Identifying individuals at increased risk of developing diabetes has assumed increasing importance with the expansion of the evidence from clinical trials on the prevention or delay of type 2 diabetes using lifestyle modification and medication. The epidemiology of prediabetes depends on the diagnostic method used. Glucose measures defining impaired glucose tolerance and impaired fasting glucose levels identify about 10% of the adults to have prediabetes, whereas glycated hemoglobin–based criteria identify a significantly lower proportion of the population. Increasingly, multifactorial risk tools are being used and cut-points set to identify approximately 15% of the population as being at high risk.

Although the state of prediabetes is defined by its role as a diabetes risk factor, it also carries a significant risk of cardiovascular disease, independent of progression to diabetes. Typical diabetic microvascular complications also occur, albeit at low rates, in prediabetes. There is evidence that both glucose-related and glucose-independent mechanisms contribute to these vascular complications. Effective preventive strategies will likely require control of glycemia, as well as other metabolic risk factors. This article reviews some of the proposed mechanisms for the vascular complications of the prediabetic state.

Prediabetes encompasses conventional diagnostic categories of impaired fasting glucose and impaired glucose tolerance but is a band of glucose concentrations and a temporal phase over a continuum extending from conventional normal glucose tolerance to overt type 2 diabetes. Insulin resistance and defective glucose sensing at the β-cell are the central pathophysiologic determinants that together cause hyperglycemia. Regardless of the cellular origin of insulin resistance, excessive tissue fat utilization is a consistent metabolic mechanism. Although genetic influences affect β-cell function, becoming overweight is the main acquired challenge to insulin action. The phenotype of prediabetes includes dyslipidemia and higher arterial blood pressure.

A rational approach to diagnosing prediabetes is essential to identify those who would benefit from entering diabetes prevention programs. Impaired fasting glucose and impaired glucose tolerance are similar in relation to their ability to identify those at risk of diabetes or cardiovascular disease; however, because they identify different segments of the at-risk population, there is value in undertaking glucose tolerance testing to ensure that both conditions can be diagnosed. Simple noninvasive diabetes risk scores offer a valuable entry point in the diagnosis of prediabetes, enabling the identification of those who need blood testing.

Primary prevention of type 2 diabetes is effective for curbing its epidemic. Lifestyle intervention has been found to be a highly effective, safe, and cost-effective method for the prevention of diabetes in high-risk persons, the benefit of which can extend for many years. Among the pharmacologic agents studied for prevention of diabetes, metformin has been found to be the safest. Interventions using drugs are less preferred because the drugs' effects tend to dissipate after their use is stopped and adverse effects may also result. The major challenge is to translate current knowledge into prevention programs at the national level.

In the United States, the costs associated with diabetes mellitus are increasing. Although people with diabetes comprise less than 6% of the US population, approximately 1 in 5 health care dollars is spent caring for people with diabetes. Healthy lifestyle interventions for the general population and intensive lifestyle and medication interventions for high-risk individuals present opportunities for diabetes prevention. This article describes the costs associated with glucose intolerance and diabetes, the effect of glucose intolerance and diabetes on the quality of life, and the cost-effectiveness of screening and primary prevention interventions for diabetes prevention.

A variety of definitions and diagnostic cutpoints have been promulgated for prediabetes without universal agreement. Professional organizations agree that current scientific evidence justifies intervention in high-risk populations for the delay or prevention of progression to diabetes. Lifestyle intervention is universally accepted as the primary intervention strategy. Secondary intervention is advocated in high-risk individuals or in the absence of a clinical response to lifestyle modification.

Peter E.H. Schwarz

Many countries are struggling to meet the health care needs of a rapidly growing number of individuals with common chronic illnesses, especially diabetes mellitus. Incorporating the evidence from prevention trials into clinical practice represents one of the major challenges for public health, and the medical community is still learning how this can best be achieved at a population level. A 4-level public health initiative has been initiated that provides guidance for establishing milestones and strategies for such a program.

Gerald S. Berenson, Mehmet Agirbasli, Quoc Manh Nguyen, Wei Chen, and Sathanur R. Srinivasan

The metabolic syndrome and adult manifestation of prediabetes and diabetes are major public health problems that begin in childhood. Prevention must be considered as a serious public health issue. Health education and health promotion of school children needs incorporation as a community effort.

Preface

Prediabetes and Diabetes Prevention

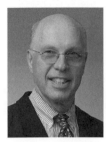

Michael Bergman, MD
Guest Editor

It is currently estimated that 57 million people (1 in 4 adults) in the Unites States have prediabetes, many of whom will develop diabetes in ensuing years unless significant modifications in lifestyle occur, including diet, weight loss, and exercise. Furthermore, a small but significant number may already be at risk for developing vascular disease. Hence, prediabetes constitutes a major international public health concern that threatens to increase dramatically given the growing prevalence of worldwide obesity. Prediabetes is also associated with considerable financial expenditure with higher rates of medical visits for hypertension, metabolic and renal complications, and general medical conditions. The national annual medical cost of prediabetes has been estimated to exceed $25 billion.[1] Since it therefore impacts considerably an already burdened healthcare system, the recently passed Affordable Care Act is opportune, as it addresses the critical need for preventive approaches to this epidemic.[2,3]

A major factor contributing to the difficulty in ascertaining who has prediabetes pertains to the way it, as diabetes per se, has been defined. As discussed in greater detail in this issue, the diagnosis of prediabetes has been predicated on absolute criteria defined by blood glucose measurements, which is one of the reasons the American Diabetes Association adopted a range of HbA1c values as a basis for identifying those at risk for developing diabetes. However, as neither glucose nor HbA1c determinations may be sufficiently sensitive to diagnose early metabolic abnormalities precisely, the practitioner requires considerable judgment in assessing these subtle conditions. Thus, defining prediabetes categorically by relatively arbitrary threshold criteria may inadvertently lead to the failure to diagnose individuals with lower glucose levels who may still be at risk for progression to diabetes or cardiovascular disease.[4]

Rather than viewing the evolving disease process as a continuum, the traditional dichotomous approach to defining metabolic entities most likely addresses only a small segment of a much larger problem and hence underestimates the considerable prevalence of this condition. One potential approach for overcoming the uncertainty associated with absolute diagnostic criteria is the use of a "personalized profile," which would

Med Clin N Am 95 (2011) xi—xiii
doi:10.1016/j.mcna.2010.11.009
0025-7125/11/$ — see front matter © 2011 Elsevier Inc. All rights reserved.

encourage early intervention in an individual demonstrating progressive deterioration of metabolic parameters, such as fasting glucose, HbA1c, and basal insulin measurements, although not yet considered abnormal on a population-based norm.[5]

Many facets of prediabetes are covered herein, including its definition (Buysschaert), epidemiology (Colagiuri), complications (Crandall), pathophysiology (Ferrannini), and diagnosis (Shaw). Furthermore, positive outcomes from large-scale prevention studies conducted in different countries, primarily with lifestyle change (Ramachandran), have translated into favorable health economic outcomes (Herman), formal treatment recommendations (Ratner), and public health initiatives in diabetes prevention (Schwarz). Finally, since obesity, metabolic syndrome, and prediabetes (as well as diabetes) occur with increasing prevalence in children and continue to evolve over a lifetime to the epidemic we witness in adults today, this perspective is also considered (Berenson).

This issue synthesizes our current knowledge of this burgeoning field. The international collaboration reflected in this work is emblematic of the global epidemic of metabolic diseases and thus provides a broad perspective on the subject matter. Furthermore, as all age groups are increasingly affected by a disease process that knows no frontiers, an incremental dialogue between adult and pediatric/adolescent physicians is therefore mandatory if we are to solve this major public health problem. As the root of adult metabolic conditions can often be traced to an earlier period, remediation is required at the earliest identifiable point in time given the indolent and continuous evolution of prediabetes and its associated risk factors.

The present work is meant for the primary care physician in particular, who sees the preponderance of individuals at risk for diabetes. However, in essence it is for every health care provider regardless of specialty, as individuals with prediabetes are often seen for unrelated medical problems. Therefore, it behooves each of us to recognize the subtle nature of the underlying metabolic disorder and intervene early and effectively. It is only through the prompt diagnosis of prediabetes and implementation of lifestyle changes very early in its denouement that we can hope to forestall the development of diabetes and its associated complications, thus decreasing the burden on the individual and on society.

The contributors to this issue are established experts in their respective fields and I am profoundly grateful to each of them for taking the time and making the effort to disseminate state-of-the-art knowledge to the readership. This has been a most rewarding collaboration. I am especially appreciative of Dr Hertzel Gerstein's advice and guidance. Dr Jesse Roth is acknowledged as well for his helpful recommendations. Finally, I would like to express my sincere thanks to Ms Rachel Glover, Editor of *Medical Clinics of North America*, for her support, insight, and professionalism, as well as to Elsevier, Inc, for agreeing to undertake this publication. Finally, I know I speak for all the authors in expressing our gratitude to each reader who ultimately affects the lives of those with prediabetes as a result of an increased awareness of this entity.

Michael Bergman, MD
Department of Medicine
Division of Endocrinology
New York University School of Medicine
345 East 37th Street, Suite 313
New York, NY 10016, USA

E-mail address:
Michael.Bergman@nyumc.org

REFERENCES

1. Zhang Y, Dall TM, Chen Y, et al. Medical cost associated with diabetes. Population Health Management 2009;12:157—63.
2. Laiteerapong N, Huang ES. Health care reform and chronic diseases: anticipating the health consequences. JAMA 2010;304:899—900.
3. Koh HK, Sebelius KG. Promoting prevention through the Affordable Care Act. Perspective. N Engl J Med 2010;363:1296—9.
4. Bergman M. Inadequacies of absolute threshold levels for diagnosing prediabetes. Commentary. Diabetes Metab Res Rev 2010;26:3—6.
5. Dankner R, Danoff A, Roth J. Can 'personalized diagnostics' promote earlier intervention for dysglycaemia? Hypothesis ready for testing. Editorial. Diabetes Metab Res Rev 2010;26:7—9.

Definition of Prediabetes

Martin Buysschaert, MD, PhD[a],*, Michael Bergman, MD[b]

KEYWORDS

• Prediabetes • Impaired fasting glucose • Glucose intolerance

Diabetes mellitus is a group of metabolic diseases characterized by hyperglycemia resulting from defects in insulin secretion, insulin action, or both.[1] Cutoff glycemic levels defining diabetes are based on the observed association between certain glucose levels and a dramatic increase in the prevalence of microvascular complications considered specific for hyperglycemia (retinopathy and nephropathy).[2] In 1979, the National Diabetes Data Group (NDDG) first introduced the concept of a metabolic state intermediate between normal glucose homeostasis and diabetes, called glucose intolerance.[3] Individuals with glucose intolerance did not meet the criteria for being diagnosed with diabetes but had glucose levels higher than those considered normal. The Expert Committee on the Diagnosis and Classification of Diabetes Mellitus extended the concept in 1997 by recognizing patients with impaired fasting glucose (IFG) in addition to those with impaired glucose tolerance (IGT).[1] Both categories (IGT and IFG) were referred to as prediabetes and are considered substantial risk factors for progression to diabetes. Moreover, microvascular complications, including retinopathy, chronic kidney disease, and neuropathy, and cardiovascular disease have been associated with prediabetes.[4–8]

The objectives of this article are to review the historical evolution of the diagnostic criteria that defined prediabetes as a condition of hyperglycemia at a lower level than diabetes and to analyze the clinical significance of prediabetes as currently diagnosed.

HISTORICAL EVOLUTION OF THE DIAGNOSTIC CRITERIA (FROM 1979 TO 2010)
From Diabetes to Glucose Intolerance: 1979 to 1997

Following the World Health Organization's (WHO) first Expert Committee Report published in 1965,[9] the NDDG in 1979 defined diabetes in adults according to 1 of

---

The authors have nothing to disclose.

a Department of Endocrinology and Diabetology, University Clinic Saint-Luc, Université Catholique de Louvain (UCL), Avenue Hippocrate 54/UCL 5474, B-1200 Brussels, Belgium
b Department of Medicine, Division of Endocrinology, New York University School of Medicine, 345 East 37th Street, Suite 313, New York, NY 10016, USA
* Corresponding author.
E-mail address: martin.buysschaert@uclouvain.be

Med Clin N Am 95 (2011) 289–297
doi:10.1016/j.mcna.2010.11.002   medical.theclinics.com
0025-7125/11/$ – see front matter © 2011 Elsevier Inc. All rights reserved.

the 3 following criteria: (1) an unequivocal elevation of plasma glucose level, with the classical signs and symptoms of polyuria, polydipsia, weight loss, and ketonuria; (2) a fasting plasma glucose (FPG) level equal to or greater than 140 mg/dL ($\geq$7.8 mmol/L) on more than 1 occasion; or (3) a 2-hour glucose level equal to or greater than 200 mg/dL ($\geq$11.1 mmol/L) and at another time between 0 and 2 hours (on more than 1 occasion) after a 75-g oral glucose tolerance test (OGTT) (**Table 1**).[3] In addition, the NDDG defined glucose intolerance as an intermediate stage character-ized by hyperglycemia but at a level lower than that qualifying for the diagnosis of dia-betes. All 3 of the following criteria had to be met before diagnosing IGT: (1) an FPG level lower than 140 mg/dL (<7.8 mmol/L), (2) a glucose value between 140 and 199 mg/dL (7.8–11.1 mmol/L) at 120 minutes after OGTT, and (3) at least 1 glucose level more than 200 mg/dL ($\geq$11.1 mmol/L) at 30, 60, and 90 minutes after the OGTT (see **Table 1**).[3] As shown in **Table 1**, the WHO stated in 1980 that glucose intolerance could be defined only by a glucose value between 140 and 199 mg/dL (8.0–11.0 mmol/L) at 120 minutes after a 75-g OGTT if the FPG level was less than 140 mg/dL (7.8 mmol/L) (ie, 2 criteria instead of 3 in the definition by NDDG).[10]

From Diabetes to Prediabetes: 1997 to 2010

The Expert Committee on the Diagnosis and Classification of Diabetes Mellitus in 1997 and the WHO in 1998 recommended that the FPG threshold be reduced from 140 mg/dL (7.8 mmol/L) to 126 mg/dL (7.0 mmol/L) for diagnosing diabetes.[1,11] The 2-hour glucose criteria after an OGTT, however, remained unchanged as equal to or greater than 200 mg/dL ($\geq$11.1 mmol/L), as well as a diagnosis was based on the presence of symptoms and measurement of a casual plasma glucose level equal to or greater than 200 mg/dL ($\geq$11.1 mmol/L) (see **Table 1**). The reduction in the FPG level was justified based on the epidemiologic observation that the cutoff of FPG level of 140 mg/dL or more defined individuals with a greater degree of hyperglycemia than did the cutoff value of the 2-hour post–glucose load. Moreover, data showing an increase in the prevalence of diabetic retinopathy beginning at approximately 126 mg/dL (7.0 mmol/L) also justified the decision.[12,13] In addition, the Expert Committee and WHO defined 2 intermediate states of abnormal glucose regulation that exist between normal glucose homeostasis and diabetes. Thus, IGT was confirmed by a 2-hour plasma glucose level between 140 and 199 mg/dL (7.8–11.1 mmol/L) after a 75-g OGTT and IFG by an FPG level between 110 and 125 mg/dL (6.1–6.9 mmol/L). The requirement for an additional glucose measurement at 30, 60, or 90 minutes to define IGT or diabetes was apparently dropped possibly to simplify the process and in view of the relationship between the 2-hour value and reti-nopathy. IFG and IGT could be observed as intermediate stages in any of the hyper-glycemic diseases reported in the Expert Committee Classification.[1]

IFG and IGT represent different pathophysiologic processes, even though these groups may overlap.[13] Although IFG and IGT are not entirely interchangeable, because FPG level alone did not always detect IGT and the 2-hour post–glucose load did not always predict IFG, both tests were useful in identifying the dysglycemic conditions.[1,11,13,14] Patients with IFG and/or IGT were considered as having a new condition referred to, for the first time, as prediabetes.[1] According to the recommen-dations of the American Diabetes Association (ADA), FPG was the preferred test for diagnosing diabetes and prediabetes because of its ease of use, acceptability to patients, and lower cost. However, OGTT could be required for further diagnosing individuals with IFG or when diabetes was still suspected despite a normal FPG level.[1] The WHO adopted most of these conclusions but stated that individuals with IFG should also undergo an OGTT to exclude IGT or diabetes.[11]

Table 1
Diagnostic criteria for diabetes and hyperglycemia at a lower level than diabetes

	NDDG (1979)[3]		WHO (1980)[10]		Expert Committee (1997)[1]		ADA (2003)[15]		ADA (2010)[20]	
	H	D	H	D	H	D	H	D	H	D
Glycemia[a]										
Fasting	<140[b] (7.8)	≥140 (7.8)	<140[b] (7.8)	≥140[c] (8.0)	110–125[d] (6.1–6.9)	≥126 (7.0)	100–125[d] (5.6–6.9)	≥126 (7.0)	100–125[d] (5.6–6.9)	≥126 (7.0)
Casual	—	—	—	≥200 (11.0)	—	≥200 (11.1)	—	≥200 (11.1)	—	≥200 (11.1)
Symptoms	—	+	—	+	—	+	—	+	—	+
OGTT (75 g)										
30 min	1 value[b] ≥200 (11.1)	1 value ≥200 (11.1)	—	—	—	—	—	—	—	—
60 min			—	—	—	—	—	—	—	—
90 min			—	—	—	—	—	—	—	—
120 min	140–199[b] (7.8–11.1)	≥200 (11.1)	140–199[b] (8.0–11.0)	≥200 (11.0)	140–199[e] (7.8–11.1)	≥200 (11.1)	140–199[e] (7.8–11.1)	≥200 (11.1)	140–199[e] (7.8–11.1)	>200 (11.1)
HbA1c (%)	—	—	—	—	—	—	—	—	5.7–6.4	≥6.5

Abbreviations: ADA, American Diabetes Association; D, diabetes; H, hyperglycemia at a lower level than diabetes.
[a] Values are expressed in mg/dL (mmol/L).
[b] Referred to as glucose intolerance.
[c] Diabetes is excluded if glucose level is <100 mg/dL (6.0 mmol/L) in the fasting state and <140 mg/dL (8.0 mmol/L) in the casual state.
[d] IFG (referred to as prediabetes). Unequivocally elevated glucose.
[e] IGT (referred to as prediabetes).

The original FPG range of 110 to 125 mg/dL (6.1–6.9 mmol/L) was further lowered in 2003 to 100 to 125 mg/dL (5.6–6.9 mmol/L) so that the population risk of developing diabetes with IFG would be similar to that with IGT.[15] Another effect of lowering the criterion for defining IFG was that individuals with IFG would more likely adopt earlier lifestyle interventions to reduce the potential risk of developing diabetes in the future.[15] Some experts did not support the latter decision,[16] and the WHO still defines IFG at the fasting glucose threshold of 110 mg/dL (6.1 mmol/L).[17] A principal reason for this decision was that the new 2003 criterion dramatically increased the number of individuals with IFG as shown by Davidson and colleagues[16] using the National Health and Nutrition Examination Survey 1999-2000 data set. Thus, the overall prevalence of IFG with the new criterion (decrease in FPG level from 110 mg/dL [6.1 mmol/L] to 100 mg/dL [5.6 mmol/L]) increased from 6.7% to 24.1%, and more than 40% of individuals older than 65 years would have IFG. Furthermore, there would be a 5-fold increase in the prevalence of IFG among individuals aged 20 to 50 years old. Individuals with IFG could potentially face the risk that insurance companies and employers would eventually take a pejorative view and consider IFG as a formal preexisting condition for diabetes, which was not supported by epidemiologic and scientific data because not everyone with prediabetes will develop diabetes.[16]

In 2010, after an extensive review of biologic and epidemiologic evidence, the glycated hemoglobin A_{1c} (HbA_{1c}) defined by a threshold level equal to or greater than 6.5% was recommended to diagnose diabetes. This recommendation was published in the ADA standards of medical care (see **Table 1**).[18–20] Diagnosis needed to be confirmed with a repeat HbA_{1c} level determination (except in symptomatic subjects with FPG>200 mg/dL). An Expert Committee pointed out that the HbA_{1c} assay had been standardized, was accurate and precise, and had several technical advantages over prevalent laboratory measurements of glucose, in particular, in terms of reduced biologic variability. It was also mentioned that the relationship between HbA_{1c} levels and the risk of microangiopathy was similar to that between the corresponding FPG and 2-hour post–glucose load levels.[19] The 1997 Expert Committee had previously reported that the prevalence of retinopathy substantially increased at HbA_{1c} values between 6.0% and 7.0%.[1] Recent data derived from DETECT-2 confirmed that the prevalence of retinopathy begins to increase with HbA_{1c} levels of 6.5%.[21]

In a study of Malay adults in Singapore, Sabanayagam and colleagues[22] similarly concluded that HbA_{1c} levels in the range from 6.6% to 7.0% were optimal for detecting microvascular complications. These investigators determined a continuous linear association between HbA_{1c} levels and microvascular complications, including retinopathy, chronic kidney disease, albuminuria, and peripheral neuropathy, without an obvious threshold effect. Despite the absence of a clear threshold effect, the HbA_{1c} range from 6.6% to 7.0% seemed to be optimal for identifying microvascular complications and could be used as well for diagnosing diabetes.

Individuals with an HbA_{1c} level between 5.7% and 6.4% would now be considered, according to the ADA, as having an increased risk for diabetes.[18–20] Thus, an FPG level of 110 mg/dL corresponds to an HbA_{1c} level of 5.6%, and an FPG level of 100 mg/dL corresponds to an HbA_{1c} level of 5.4%. As risk presents as a continuum, HbA_{1c} values between 6.0% and 6.5% represent the greatest risk for progression to diabetes for which preventive measures might be implemented. In individuals with HbA_{1c} levels lower than 6.0%, the presence of other risk factors for diabetes in addition to HbA_{1c} levels should be taken into account in determining when to initiate medical interventions.

The strategy of using the HbA_{1c} level for identifying individuals with diabetes or at (high) risk for diabetes has, however, been challenged, in particular by Bloomgarden,[23] based on the observation that several medical conditions are associated with alterations in the relationship between mean glycemia and HbA_{1c} levels. Limitations of the HbA_{1c} determination include specific hemoglobinopathies that interfere with older HbA_{1c} assays (eg, fetal hemoglobin falsely increases and sickle cell hemoglobin/hemoglobin C lowers HbA_{1c} levels). Diseases changing the turnover of red blood cells, such as hemolysis, shortened erythrocyte life, cirrhosis, acute or chronic blood loss, or transfusions, may also lead to abnormally low HbA_{1c} levels. Patients with these conditions could, therefore, risk the possibility of a false-negative diagnosis. In contrast, the use of HbA_{1c} levels could also lead to overdiagnosis of diabetes (ie, false-positive diagnosis) among the elderly, subjects with iron deficiency, or individuals genetically predisposed to greater levels of hemoglobin glycation. Black individuals have higher HbA_{1c} levels than white individuals across the continuum of glycemia, and larger differences are associated with more severe glucose intolerance.[24,25] In these patients and during pregnancy, traditional diagnostic tests based on glucose criteria, and not HbA_{1c}, should be used as in other conditions.[25] The use of alternate methods for diagnosing dysglycemic conditions also applies to settings where standardized HbA_{1c} methods are unavailable.

In summary, it is reasonable to consider, as stated by the ADA, an HbA_{1c} range of 5.7% to 6.4% for identifying individuals at (high) risk for diabetes, to whom the term prediabetes can be applied, and values higher than 6.5% can be used for diagnosing diabetes.[20] However, using these HbA_{1c} criteria, Cowie and colleagues[26] detected a substantially lower prevalence of "high risk for diabetes" or diabetes than that detected with the glucose criteria. The crude prevalence of total diabetes in adults aged 20 years or older was 9.6% (20.4 million), of which 19.0% was undiagnosed. Another 3.5% of adults (7.4 million) were at high risk for diabetes (HbA_{1c}, 6.0% to <6.5%). Prevalences of undiagnosed diabetes and high risk of diabetes were, respectively, one-third and one-tenth that using the glucose criteria. Prevalences were disproportionately high in the elderly and more than 2 times higher in non-Hispanic blacks and Mexican Americans compared with non-Hispanic whites. A high risk for diabetes was more than 2 times higher in non-Hispanic blacks than in non-Hispanic whites and Mexican Americans.

As already described, factors unrelated to glucose control, such as hemoglobin glycation or red blood cell survival, may differ among racial/ethnic groups, which may explain the disproportionately greater prevalence of undiagnosed and high risk of diabetes observed in these populations.[26] Furthermore, as also noted previously, HbA_{1c} concentrations can be misleading in certain medical conditions, and therefore, diagnosis of prediabetes should be based exclusively on the glucose criteria in these circumstances. **Box 1** summarizes the current criteria for diagnosing individuals at increased risk for diabetes (prediabetes) according to the ADA clinical practice recommendations.[20]

CONSIDERATIONS FOR THE CURRENT DEFINITION OF PREDIABETES (INCREASED RISK FOR DIABETES)

Prediabetes (IFG and/or IGT) should be viewed as a stage in the natural history of disordered glucose metabolism rather than as a distinctive clinical entity representing an interim condition and as a risk factor presaging (1) the development of diabetes (increased risk for diabetes) and (2) an increase in cardiovascular and possibly microvascular complications.

The transition from prediabetes to diabetes may take many years but may also be rapid.[27,28] Current estimates indicate that most individuals (up to 70%) with

---

Box 1
Criteria for prediabetes (categories of increased risk for diabetes[a])

IFG

    FPG: 100 to 125 mg/dL (5.6–6.9 mmol/L)

IGT

    FPG less than 100 mg/dL (5.6 mmol/L)

    Two-hour plasma glucose level after 75-g OGTT: 140 to 199 mg/dL (7.8–11.0 mmol/L)

    HbA$_{1c}$: 5.7% to 6.4%

[a] For all 3 tests, the ADA states that risk is continuous, extending below the lower limit of the range and becoming disproportionately greater at higher ends of the range.
Adapted from The International Expert Committee. International Expert Committee Report on the role of the A$_{1c}$ assay in the diagnosis of diabetes. Diabetes Care 2009;32:1327–34.

---

prediabetes eventually develop diabetes. The incidence is highest in individuals with combined IFG and IGT and similar in those with isolated IFG or IGT.[27] The average risk of developing diabetes is about 5% to 10% per year in individuals with IFG or IGT compared with approximately 0.7% per year in normoglycemic individuals.[29]

Importantly, the progression to diabetes may follow a continuum and occur at glucose and HbA$_{1c}$ values lower than those meeting the current definition of IFG.[30] Shaw and colleagues[31] and, more recently, Nichols and colleagues[32] showed that the risk of diabetes increased with an FPG level even within the currently accepted normal range. Thus, an FPG level of 90 to 94 mg/dL (5.0–5.2 mmol/L) conferred a 49% greater risk of developing diabetes when compared with a level lower than 85 mg/dL (4.7 mmol/L). The hazard ratio (HR) for diabetes was 2.33 (95% confidence interval [CI], 1.95–2.79) for subjects with glucose levels of 95 to 99 mg/dL.[26] Abdul-Ghani and colleagues[33] reported that an increase in the 2-hour post–glucose load value in the normal range was also associated with an increase in the incidence of type 2 diabetes as were 1-hour post–glucose load values exceeding 150 mg/dL.

Based on numerous longitudinal studies, prediabetes (IGT and IFG) has also been associated with an increased risk for cardiovascular events, with IGT being a slightly stronger risk predictor.[1,4,30] IFG and IGT are frequently associated with other cardiovascular risk factors, such as obesity, in particular abdominal or visceral obesity; dyslipidemia with high triglyceride levels and/or low high-density lipoprotein cholesterol levels; and hypertension. However, there is substantial evidence that cardiovascular risk increases continually with increasing FPG levels alone and that the progressive relationship between glucose levels and cardiovascular risk also extends below the prediabetic threshold. Hoogwerf and colleagues[34] and others[35,36] showed that the relationship between glucose and coronary heart disease risk is also continuous and graded across the range of nondiabetic glucose values independent of traditional risk factors. Moreover, the recent data of Selvin and colleagues[30] confirmed this observation by demonstrating that the HbA$_{1c}$ level was strongly associated with cardiovascular risk in a population of nondiabetic adults. The multivariable-adjusted HRs (with 95% CIs) were 1.78 (1.48–2.15) and 1.95 (1.53–2.48) for HbA$_{1c}$ values between 5.5% and 6.0% and between 6.0% and 6.5%, respectively. Prediabetes is also associated with the development of microangiopathy as observed in particular in the Diabetes Prevention Program, which demonstrated that 7.9% of participants with IGT had findings consistent with diabetic retinopathy.[5]

From a practical perspective, the use of absolute glucose threshold values for prediabetes, below which there are few complications and above which the prevalence of complications increases incrementally, has resulted in defining these entities categorically, hence facilitating classification. Moreover, a diagnosis of prediabetes also has considerable implications with regard to the potential development of diabetes and cardiovascular (and possibly microangiopathic) complications and also for treatment. However, a categorical classification fails to acknowledge the importance of a principle of continuum of risk for developing diabetes and related complications previously commented on by Bergman.[19,37–39] Therefore, even if seemingly arbitrary cutoff values are inevitably required for clinical use and classification, the concept of continuous risk suggests that glucose and HbA$_{1c}$ levels lower than those currently defining prediabetes should encourage the practitioner to engage patients in prevention counseling. Intervention is particularly warranted when other conventional cardiovascular risk factors are present.

REFERENCES

1. The Expert Committee on the Diagnosis and Classification of Diabetes Mellitus. Report of the Expert Committee on the Diagnosis and Classification of Diabetes Mellitus. Diabetes Care 1997;20:1183–97.
2. Pettitt DJ, Knowler WC, Lisse JR, et al. Development of retinopathy and proteinuria in relation to plasma-glucose concentrations in Pima Indians. Lancet 1980;2: 1050–2.
3. National Diabetes Data Group. Classification and diagnosis of diabetes mellitus and other categories of glucose intolerance. Diabetes 1979;28:1039–57.
4. Coutinho M, Gerstein HC, Wang Y, et al. The relationship between glucose and incident cardiovascular events. Diabetes Care 1999;22:233–40.
5. Diabetes Prevention Program Research Group. The prevalence of retinopathy in impaired glucose tolerance and recent-onset diabetes in the Diabetes Prevention Program. Diabet Med 2007;24:137–44.
6. Sumner CJ, Sheth S, Griffin JW, et al. The spectrum of neuropathy in diabetes and impaired glucose tolerance. Neurology 2003;60:108–11.
7. Plantinga LC, Crews DC, Coresh J, et al. Prevalence of chronic kidney disease in US adults with undiagnosed diabetes or prediabetes. Clin J Am Soc Nephrol 2010;5:673–82.
8. Cheng YL, Gregg EW, Geiss LS. Association of A1C and fasting plasma glucose levels with diabetic retinopathy prevalence in the U.S. population. Diabetes Care 2009;32:2027–32.
9. World Health Organization Expert Committee on Diabetes Mellitus. Second WHO Technical Report, Series 310. Geneva (Switzerland): World Health Organization; 1965.
10. World Health Organization. Diabetes mellitus: report of a WHO Study Group. Technical Report, Series 727. Geneva (Switzerland): World Health Organization; 1980.
11. Alberti KG, Zimmet PZ. Definition, diagnosis and classification of diabetes mellitus and its complications. Part 1: diagnosis and classification of diabetes mellitus provisional report of a WHO consultation. Diabet Med 1998;15(7):539–53.
12. Engelgau MM, Thompson TJ, Herman WH, et al. Comparison of fasting and 2-hour glucose and HbA$_{1c}$ levels for diagnosing diabetes. Diagnostic criteria and performance revisited. Diabetes Care 1997;20:785–91.

13. Borch-Johnsen K. IGT and IFG. Time for revision? Diabet Med 2002;19:707.
14. Unwin N, Shaw J, Zimmet P, et al. Impaired glucose tolerance and impaired fasting glycaemia: the current status on definition and intervention. Diabet Med 2002; 19:708–23.
15. The Expert Committee on the Diagnosis and Classification of Diabetes Mellitus. Follow-up report on the diagnosis of diabetes mellitus. Diabetes Care 2003;26: 3160–7.
16. Davidson MB, Landsman PB, Alexander CM. Lowering the criterion for impaired fasting glucose will not provide clinical benefit. Diabetes Care 2003;26:3329–30.
17. World Health Organization/International Diabetes Federation. Definition and diagnosis of diabetes mellitus and intermediate hyperglycaemia: report of the WHO/IDF consultation. Available at: http://www.who.int/diabetes/publications/ Definition%20and%20diagnosis%20of%20diabetes_new.pdf. Accessed April 28, 2008.
18. Saudek CD, Herman WH, Sacks DB, et al. A new look at screening and diagnosing diabetes mellitus. J Clin Endocrinol Metab 2008;93(7):2447–53.
19. The International Expert Committee. International Expert Committee Report on the role of the A_{1C} assay in the diagnosis of diabetes. Diabetes Care 2009;32: 1327–34.
20. American Diabetes Association. Standards of medical care in diabetes—2010. Diabetes Care 2010;33(Suppl 1):S11–61.
21. The DETECT-2 Collaboration Writing Group, Colagiuri S, Lee CM, et al. Glycemic thresholds for diabetes-specific retinopathy: implications for diagnosis criteria for diabetes. Diabetes Care 2010. [Epub ahead of print].
22. Sabanayagam L, Liew G, Tai ES, et al. Relationship between glycated haemoglobin and microvascular complications: is there a natural cut-off point for the diagnosis of diabetes? Diabetologia 2009;52:1279–89.
23. Bloomgarden Z. A_{1C}: recommendations, debates and questions. Diabetes Care 2009;32:141–7.
24. Ziemer DC, Kolm P, Weintraub WS, et al. Glucose-independent, black-white differences in hemoglobin A_{1C} levels. Ann Intern Med 2010;152:770–7.
25. Herman WH, Cohen RM. Hemoglobin A_{1C}: teaching a new dog old tricks. Ann Intern Med 2010;152:815–7.
26. Cowie CC, Rust KF, Byrd-Holt DD, et al. Prevalence of diabetes and high risk for diabetes using A1C criteria in the U.S. population in 1988-2006. Diabetes Care 2010;33:562–8.
27. Nathan DM, Davidson MB, DeFronzo RA, et al. Impaired fasting glucose and impaired glucose tolerance. Diabetes Care 2007;30:753–9.
28. Ferrannini E, Nannipieri M, Williams K, et al. Mode of onset of type 2 diabetes from normal or impaired glucose tolerance. Diabetes 2004;53:160–5.
29. Aroda VR, Ratner R. Approach to the patient with prediabetes. J Clin Endocrinol Metab 2008;93(9):3259–65.
30. Selvin E, Steffes MW, Zhu H, et al. Glycated hemoglobin, diabetes and cardiovascular risk in nondiabetic adults. N Engl J Med 2010;362:800–11.
31. Shaw JE, Zimmet PZ, Hodge AM, et al. Impaired fasting glucose: how low should it go? Diabetes Care 2000;23:34–9.
32. Nichols GA, Hillier TA, Brown JB. Normal fasting plasma glucose and risk of type 2 diabetes diagnosis. Am J Med 2008;121:519–24.
33. Abdul-Ghani MA, Stern MP, Lyssenko V, et al. Minimal contribution of fasting hyperglycemia to the incidence of type 2 diabetes in subjects with normal 2-h plasma glucose. Diabetes Care 2010;33:557–61.

34. Hoogwerf BJ, Spreche DL, Pearce GL, et al. Blood glucose concentrations ≤125 mg/dl and coronary heart disease risk. Am J Cardiol 2002;89:556–9.
35. Khaw KT, Wareham N, Luben R, et al. Glycated hemoglobin, diabetes, and mortality in men in Norfolk cohort of European Prospective Investigation of Cancer and Nutrition (EPIC-Norfolk). BMJ 2001;322:1–6.
36. Barrett-Connor E, Wingard DL. "Normal" blood glucose and coronary risk. BMJ 2001;322:5–6.
37. Bergman M. Inadequacies of absolute threshold levels for diagnosing prediabetes [editorial]. Diabetes Metab Res Rev 2009;26:7–9.
38. Bergman M. A review of prediabetes and implications of current threshold levels. Louvain Med 2009;128:S15–24.
39. Borg R, Kuenen JC, Carstensen B, et al. Real-life glycemic profiles in non-diabetic individuals with low fasting glucose and normal HbA_{1c}: the A1C-Derived Average Glucose (ADAG) Study. Diabetologia 2010;53:1608–11.

Epidemiology of Prediabetes

Stephen Colagiuri, MB BS, FRACP

KEYWORDS

- Prediabetes • Prevalence • Risk assessment • Type 2 diabetes

---

Detecting individuals at risk of future diseases and implementing programs to reduce risk of progression to disease is a fundamental objective of reducing the burden of conditions such as diabetes. In addition, prevention of diabetes also offers the opportunity to reduce the risk of cardiovascular disease, which is the major cause of premature death and chronic disability.

High-risk states for the future development of diabetes have been officially recognized for many years and have been given different names. In 1965, one of the first formal definitions was proposed by a World Health Organization (WHO) Expert Committee, which recommended the term borderline diabetes.[1] At that time prediabetes was considered a retrospective diagnosis and was applied to people with normal glucose tolerance who later developed diabetes. Over the years, the term prediabetes has evolved and now covers various definitions. Consequently, the epidemiology of prediabetes depends on the definition used.

EPIDEMIOLOGY OF PREDIABETES ACCORDING TO DEFINITION
Intermediate Hyperglycemia

The most common definition of prediabetes refers to impaired glucose tolerance (IGT) and impaired fasting glucose (IFG). IGT and IFG were conceived to define categories of glycemia associated with an increased risk of developing diabetes.[2–5] In an epidemiologic framework, IGT and IFG are standardized ways of describing the prevalence of intermediate hyperglycemia in different populations at any one time or in the same population over time. These categories have proved useful in describing the extent of the disease burden in a population and for engaging policy makers.[6]

Prevalence
Numerous epidemiologic studies from many countries have documented the prevalence of IGT. These prevalence data are summarized in the International Diabetes Federation's (IDF's) *Diabetes Atlas*.[7] It is estimated that some 344 million people

---

Financial disclosure: None relevant.
Boden Institute of Obesity, Nutrition and Exercise, University of Sydney, K25 Medical Foundation Building, New South Wales 2006, Australia
E-mail address: Stephen.colagiuri@sydney.edu.au

Med Clin N Am 95 (2011) 299–307
doi:10.1016/j.mcna.2010.11.003
0025-7125/11/$ – see front matter © 2011 Elsevier Inc. All rights reserved.

medical.theclinics.com

worldwide, or 7.9% in the age group of 20 to 79 years, have IGT in 2010, the vast majority of who live in low- and middle-income countries. By 2030, the number of people with IGT is projected to increase to 472 million, or 8.4% of the adult population. The prevalence of IGT varies by IDF region as shown in **Table 1**.

However, these prevalence data may already be outdated. Recently published data from a large population-based sample of more than 45,000 people 20 years and older in China found rates of IGT and IFG of 15.5%, double the rate reported in the *Diabetes Atlas*. Rates of prediabetes were slightly higher in rural than in urban areas, the opposite of what has been reported in the past. The implication of these figures for the future burden of diabetes is of particular concern.[8]

IGT is typically more common in women than in men, and the prevalence varies across age groups. In the Diabetes Epidemiology: Collaborative analysis of Diagnostic criteria in Europe (DECODE) study, the prevalence of isolated IGT increased from 2.9% in 30- to 39-year-old men to 15.1% in 70- to 79-year-old men and from 4.5% in 30- to 39-year-old women to 16.9% in 70- to 79-year old women.[9] A similar pattern was observed in Asian populations, with the prevalence of IGT increasing with age up to 70 to 89 years. However, some populations were different. For example, in India, where the overall prevalence of IGT is higher, there is not much change with age.[10]

The IDF has not published prevalence data for IFG. In addition, the situation with IFG is more complex than that with IGT because at present there are 2 definitions in use, the WHO definition of fasting plasma glucose level being 6.1 to 6.9 mmol/L (110–125 mg/dL)[11] and the American Diabetes Association (ADA) definition of fasting plasma glucose level being 5.6 to 6.9 mmol/L (100–125 mg/dL).[12]

The issue is further complicated in that using only fasting plasma glucose levels means that some people defined as having IFG will have other abnormalities of glucose tolerance, including diabetes. The DECODE data show that in European people with a fasting plasma glucose level of 6.1 to 6.9 mmol/L (110–125 mg/dL), 64.8% have isolated IFG, 28.6% have IGT, and 6.6% actually have diabetes based on the 2-hour post–glucose-load plasma glucose level.[9] Similarly, Diabetes Epidemiology: Collaborative Analysis Of Diagnostic Criteria in Asia (DECODA) data show that among Asian people with a fasting plasma glucose level of 6.1 to 6.9 mmol/L (110–125 mg/dL) alone, 45.9% have isolated IFG, 35.2% have IGT, and 18.9% have diabetes.[10]

Although the overall prevalence of WHO-defined IFG is of the order of 5%, prevalence rates vary among populations and across different age groups. IFG is typically more common in men than in women. Prevalence of isolated IFG increased in the DECODE study from 5.2% in 30- to 39-year-old men up to 10.1% in 50- to 59-year-old men and then decreased to 3.2% in 80- to 89-year-old men, whereas in women, the prevalence increased from 2.6% in 30 to 39 year olds to 5.9% in 70- to 79-year-old

Table 1
World estimates of IGT (adjusted to the world population) by the IDF region

Region	Prevalence
Africa	8.1%
Europe	8.9%
Middle East and North Africa	8.2%
North America and Caribbean	10.4%
South and Central America	7.5%
South East Asia	6.2%
Western Pacific	7.7%

individuals.[9] In Asian populations, the prevalence of isolated IFG generally increases with age, although again the Indian population is different with little change with age.[10]

In 2003, the ADA revised the cut-point for IFG to 5.6 mmol/L (100 mg/dL).[12] This revision was based on receiver operator curve (ROC) analyses of Pima Indian, Mauritius, San Antonio, and Hoorn study data, which identified the baseline fasting plasma glucose levels that maximized sensitivity and specificity for predicting diabetes over a 5-year period. However, the WHO in its 2006 review concluded that taking into account a broad range of factors, there was no compelling reason to lower the fasting plasma glucose levels used to define IFG.[11]

Several studies have reported a 2- to 3-fold increase in IFG prevalence using the ADA recommended criterion as opposed to the WHO-defined criterion, highlighted by data from the DETECT-2 study.[13] The prevalence of IFG increases from 11.8% to 37.6% in Denmark, from 10.6% to 37.6% in India, and from 9.5% to 28.5% in the United States for WHO- and ADA-defined criteria for IFG, respectively. Such increases have major consequences in countries such as India and China where the number of people with IFG in the 40 to 64 year age range would increase by 13 million and 20 million, respectively, using the ADA definition of IFG.

Natural history
As measures of future risk of diabetes, IGT and IFG identify a group of people at higher risk. The annualized relative risk of a person with IGT progressing to diabetes is increased 6-fold when compared with people with normal glucose tolerance.[14] This relative risk is 12-fold higher in people with both IFG and IGT. The annualized relative risk of people with isolated IFG progressing to diabetes is 4.7-fold compared with people with normal glucose tolerance.[14]

The risk of people with IGT and/or IFG developing diabetes is not uniform. An analysis of 6 prospective studies showed that the incidence rates of diabetes in people with IGT ranged from 35.8 to 87.3 per 1000 person-years.[15] In addition, the rates vary according to the 2-hour plasma glucose level, with the risk of future diabetes increasing with the glucose distribution in people with IGT. For example Gabir and colleagues[16] showed that the 5-year cumulative incidence for new diabetes in Pima Indians was 17% for those with a 2-hour plasma glucose level of 7.8 to 9.2 mmol/L (140–166 mg/dL) and 39% for those with a 2-hour plasma glucose level of 9.3 to 11.0 mmol/L (167–198 mg/dL).

The same also applies for IFG. Forouhi and colleagues[17] examined the magnitude of the association between different thresholds for IFG and future diabetes. Overall, the magnitude of the association between diabetes and IFG is greater when defined by a fasting plasma glucose level of 6.1 to 6.9 mmol/L (110–125 mg/dL) than 5.6 to 6.0 mmol/L (100–108 mg/dL). For example, in the Data from an Epidemiologic Study on the Insulin Resistance Syndrome (DESIR) study, the diabetes incidence rates per 1000 person-years for the fasting plasma glucose level categories of less than 5.6 mmol/L (100 mg/dL), 5.6 to 6.0 mmol/L (100–108 mg/dL), and 6.1 to 6.9 mmol/L (110–124 mg/dL) were, respectively, 1.8, 5.7, and 43.2 in men and 0.7, 6.2, and 54.7 in women.[18] In the Mauritius study, the 5-year incidence of diabetes was in the order of 15% for a fasting plasma glucose level of 5.5 to 5.7 mmol/L (99–103 mg/dL) compared with 30% for a fasting plasma glucose level of 6.1 to 6.9 mmol/L (110–124 mg/dL).[19]

Although IGT and IFG denote a state of increased risk of progression to diabetes, many revert to normal glucose tolerance. Data from the Mauritius study indicated that of those with IGT at baseline, 30% reverted to normal, 35% continued to have IGT, 5% developed IFG, and 30% developed diabetes over the 11-year follow-up period.[19]

Reproducibility
The reproducibility of IGT with retesting within 6 weeks is only moderate. On retesting individuals with IFG within 6 weeks, the proportion of patients classified as having IFG on the first test and on retesting is approximately 50% to 60%, with the majority being reclassified as normal and less than 10% as having diabetes with repeat testing.[14] Similarly, the proportion of people classified with IGT on the first oral glucose tolerance test (OGTT) and on retesting ranged from 33% to 48%, with 39% to 46% being reclassified as normal and 6% to 13% as having diabetes on repeat testing.[14]

Increased risk of cardiovascular disease
While IGT was initially defined as a category of glycemia associated with an increased risk of developing diabetes, it is increasingly recognized as being associated with an increased risk of premature mortality and cardiovascular disease, although the risk of latter is less than that of developing diabetes. The annualized relative risk for all-cause mortality was 1.5-fold higher in people with IGT compared with people with normal glucose tolerance. The relative risk of a fatal cardiovascular outcome was 1.7-fold higher for people with IGT and 1.2-fold higher for those with IFG.[14]

As with diabetes risk, the risk of cardiovascular disease increases with increasing fasting and 2-hour plasma glucose levels across the nondiabetic range, without an obvious threshold. Both a linear[20,21] and a J-shaped relationship[22,23] have been reported for the increase in cardiovascular events and mortality with postchallenge plasma glucose level in the nondiabetic range.

Glycated Hemoglobin

Glycated hemoglobin (HbA_{1c}) has been recommended by an International Expert Committee as a diagnostic criterion for diabetes,[24] with an HbA_{1c} level greater than or equal to 6.5% being diagnostic of diabetes. Whereas this recommendation has been adopted by the ADA,[25] the WHO is currently considering the issue and is yet to make an official statement.

The International Expert Committee did not recommend a level of HbA_{1c} that could be used to diagnose states of intermediate hyperglycemia but recognized that levels of HbA_{1c} just less than 6.5% may indicate increased risk of future diabetes. This Committee recommended that people with an HbA_{1c} between 6.0% and 6.5% were at a particularly high risk and could therefore be considered for a diabetes prevention intervention.[24] Subsequently, the ADA has recommended that individuals with an HbA_{1c} of 5.7% to 6.4% be considered at increased risk for diabetes and cardiovascular disease and receive counseling to lower their risk.[25]

Because this is a very recent recommendation, there are limited data on the prevalence of HbA_{1c}-defined prediabetes. However, it is clear that the different categories of intermittent hyperglycemia (IGT, IFG, and HbA_{1c}) do not detect the same groups of individuals as being at high risk.

Based on 2003–2006 US National Health and Nutrition Examination Survey (NHANES) data, 3.5% of people 20 years and older (7.4 million individuals) were at a high risk for diabetes defined by an HbA_{1c} of 6.0% to 6.4%. Prevalence increased significantly with age (3.7% in those aged 40–59 years and 7.1% in those aged 60–74 years) but did not differ by gender. Prevalence using this HbA_{1c} criterion was about one-tenth that using fasting plasma glucose/2-hour glucose criteria (29.0% combined, 25.2% IFG, and 13.6% IGT).[26] In addition, racial differences were noted, with the proportion at high risk for diabetes in people aged 65 years and older being higher in non-Hispanic blacks (13.2%) than in non-Hispanic whites (7.7%) and Mexican Americans (8.3%). These racial/ethnic differences in the prevalence of high risk of diabetes are disproportionately greater using

HbA_{1c}, which, in part, may be explained by the now well-recognized black-white difference in the relationship between blood glucose levels and HbA_{1c}, with black persons having a higher level than white persons across the full spectrum of glycemia, with the difference increasing with worsening glucose tolerance.[27]

The 1999–2006 NHANES data were analyzed to determine the percentage and number of US adults without diabetes classified as having prediabetes by HbA_{1c} of 5.7% to 6.4% and ADA-defined IFG. The prevalence of prediabetes was 12.6% by the HbA_{1c} criterion and 28.2% by the fasting glucose criterion, with 7.7% having prediabetes according to both definitions. HbA_{1c} alone would reclassify 37.6 million Americans with IFG as not having prediabetes and 8.9 million without IFG as having prediabetes (46.5 million reclassified).[28]

Natural history

HbA_{1c} predicts the development of diabetes. Pradhan and colleagues[29] measured HbA_{1c} at baseline in a cohort of 26,563 US females aged 45 years or older without known diabetes or vascular disease. During a median follow-up of 10.1 years, 1238 cases of diabetes and 684 cardiovascular events occurred. After multivariate adjustment, HbA_{1c} was a strong predictor of diabetes but not cardiovascular disease. The adjusted relative risks for incident diabetes in HbA_{1c} categories of less than 5.0%, 5.0% to 5.4%, 5.5% to 5.9%, 6.0% to 6.4%, 6.5% to 6.9%, and greater than or equal to 7.0% were 1.0, 2.9, 12.1, 29.3, 28.2, and 81.2, respectively.

Selvin and colleagues[30] analyzed data from the Atherosclerosis Risk in Communities cohort to assess the relationship of HbA_{1c} and incident diabetes, coronary heart disease, and stroke. The cumulative incidence over 15 years of diagnosed diabetes was 6%, 12%, 21%, 44%, and 79% among participants with an HbA_{1c} of less than 5.0%, 5.0 to less than 5.5%, 5.5% to less than 6.0%, 6.0% to less than 6.5%, and greater than or equal to 6.5%, respectively. The HbA_{1c} at baseline was associated with newly diagnosed diabetes and cardiovascular outcomes. For HbA_{1c} values of less than 5.0%, 5.0% to less than 5.5%, 5.5% to less than 6.0%, 6.0% to less than 6.5%, and greater than or equal to 6.5%, the multivariable-adjusted hazard ratios for diagnosed diabetes were 0.52, 1.00 (reference), 1.86, 4.48, and 16.47, respectively. For coronary heart disease, the hazard ratios were 0.96, 1.00 (reference), 1.23, 1.78, and 1.95, respectively. The hazard ratios for stroke were similar.

RISK SCORES

There have been 2 main reasons for the recent focus on developing risk scores to identify individuals at high risk of developing diabetes. First, although the current glycemic cut-points used to define prediabetes seem to be operationally adequate, the risk of future diabetes begins to increase at levels below the ranges defined by these somewhat arbitrary cut-points. Defining specific levels for intermediate hyperglycemia may not be the most appropriate way of defining future risk of diabetes or cardiovascular disease. Consequently, the 2006 WHO report concluded that a risk score combining known risk factors, which includes a measure of glycemia would seem a more logical approach to predicting risk of diabetes.[11]

Second, the emergence of evidence from clinical trials showing that prevention of type 2 diabetes with lifestyle intervention is possible has increased the desirability of having simple methods for identifying high-risk individuals who might benefit from preventive interventions. Identification of such individuals through invasive blood tests, such as the OGTT, is not feasible at the population level. These risk tools can be used to identify people at high risk who are offered a lifestyle program or can be the initial step in a 2-step screening procedure in which the risk tool is used to identify people who require further testing.

Several risk tools have been developed across different populations. One of the first tool for predicting diabetes was Finnish Diabetes Risk Score (FINDRISC),[31] and subsequently other tools have been developed in different countries, which are being used in community-based prevention projects.[32–37] Variables included in determining risk are generally similar and typically include age, a measure of weight (body mass index, waist circumference), history of hypertension and high blood glucose levels (including gestational diabetes), and physical activity. These risk scores typically have sensitivities and specificities around 75% to 80%, depending on the cutoff value used to define increased risk.

The percentage of the population identified as being at high risk based on risk tool assessment entirely depends on the cut-point used. The setting of the cut-point is influenced by many factors, including sensitivity, specificity, and positive predictive value (PPV). Equally important from a public health and health system perspective is the proportion of the population identified and the feasibility and cost of a screening and intervention program. Consequently, most commonly the risk score cut-point is set in order to identify approximately 15% of the target population as being at high risk. For example, with the Australian risk tool for predicting the development of diabetes, Australian Type 2 Diabetes Risk Assessment Tool (AUSDRISK), a score of 12 or more had a sensitivity of 74.0%, specificity of 67.7%, and PPV of 12.7 and identified 20% of the population as being at high risk, whereas the corresponding results for a score of 15 or more were 54.3%, 83.1%, 16.7%, and 16.5%.[33]

Although these risk scores were developed to predict incident diabetes, they are also useful for identifying undiagnosed diabetes and intermediate hyperglycemia. Using a cut-point of 11 or more, the FINDRISC tool had an area under the ROC of 0.65 and a sensitivity of 45.6% and specificity of 75.4% in men and a sensitivity of 53.4% and specificity of 65.8% in women for intermediate hyperglycemia. In addition to identifying individuals at high risk of type 2 diabetes, FINDRISC identified individuals at increased risk of cardiovascular disease as illustrated by its ability to identify individuals with National Cholesterol Education Program-defined metabolic syndrome.[38]

SUMMARY

Identification of individuals at increased risk for developing diabetes has assumed increasing importance with expansion of the evidence base from clinical trials on the prevention or delay of type 2 diabetes using lifestyle modification or medication. This approach is now an integral part of strategies for reducing the diabetes burden. Importantly, this approach has implications for maintenance of good health in an individual and from a population and public health perspective because health systems around the world struggle to contain the epidemic of chronic diseases.

There are several ways of identifying individuals at high risk of diabetes, each with their advantages and disadvantages in relation to their ability to accurately quantify risk and their practical application. Consequently, the number of individuals identified at high risk will vary with the method used. Also, a particular individual may be classified as being at high risk by one method but not by another. Although all methods perform satisfactorily at a population level, many people who will never develop diabetes will be identified as being at increased risk. However, offering these individuals a lifestyle modification program is unlikely to do harm and provides potential benefit. Perhaps of greater concern is that some who will develop diabetes will be classified as not being at increased risk and will be inappropriately reassured. This situation should be addressed by ongoing research into improving the risk assessment methods.

REFERENCES

1. World Health Organization. Diabetes mellitus: report of a WHO expert committee. Geneva (Switzerland): World Health Organisation; 1965. (Tech. Rep. Ser., no. 310). Available at: http://www.who.int/diabetes/publications/Definition%20and%20diagnosis%20of%20diabetes_new.pdf. Accessed October 9, 2010.
2. Classification and diagnosis of diabetes mellitus and other categories of glucose intolerance. National Diabetes Data Group. Diabetes 1979;28:1039–57.
3. World Health Organization. Expert Committee on Diabetes Mellitus. Geneva (Switzerland): World Health Organisation; 1980. (Tech. Rep. Ser., no. 646). Available at: http://www.who.int/diabetes/publications/Definition%20and%20diagnosis%20of%20diabetes_new.pdf. Accessed October 9, 2010.
4. National Diabetes Data Group, Classification and diagnosis of diabetes mellitus and other categories of glucose intolerance. Diabetes Care 1997;20:1183–97.
5. World Health Organization. Definition, diagnosis and classification of diabetes mellitus and its complications: report of a WHO consultation. Part 1: diagnosis and classification of diabetes mellitus. Geneva (Switzerland): World Health Organisation; 1999.
6. Colagiuri S, Borch-Johnsen K, Wareham NJ. Back to the future – Do IGT and IFG have value as clinical entities? Diabetes Res Clin Pract 2008;81:131–3.
7. Diabetes atlas. 4th edition. Brussels (Belgium): International Diabetes Federation; 2009. Available at: http://www.diabetesatlas.org/. Accessed October 9, 2010.
8. Yang W, Lu J, Weng J, et al, for the China National Diabetes and Metabolic Disorders Study Group. Prevalence of diabetes among men and women in China. N Engl J Med 2010;362:1090–101.
9. DECODE Study Group. Age- and sex-specific prevalences of diabetes and impaired glucose regulation in 13 European Cohorts. Diabetes Care 2003;26:61–9.
10. Qiao Q, Hu G, Tuomilehto J, et al. DECODA Study Group. Age- and sex-specific prevalence of diabetes and impaired glucose regulation in 11 Asian Cohorts. Diabetes Care 2003;26:1770–80.
11. World Health Organization. Definition and diagnosis of diabetes mellitus and intermediate hyperglycemia. Geneva (Switzerland): World Health Organisation; 2006. Available at: http://www.who.int/diabetes/publications/Definition%20and%20diagnosis%20of%20diabetes_new.pdf. Accessed October 9, 2010.
12. Genuth S, Alberti KG, Bennett P, et al, The Expert Committee on the Diagnosis and Classification of Diabetes Mellitus. Follow-up report on the diagnosis of diabetes mellitus. Diabetes Care 2003;26:3160–7.
13. Borch-Johnsen K, Colagiuri S, Balkau B, et al. Creating a pandemic of prediabetes: the proposed new diagnostic criteria for impaired fasting glycaemia. Diabetologia 2004;47:1396–402.
14. McMaster University Evidence Based Practice Center. Diagnosis, prognosis and treatment of impaired glucose tolerance and impaired fasting glucose, Evidence Report 128. Available at: http://www.ahrq.gov. Accessed October 9, 2010.
15. Edelstein SL, Knowler WC, Bain RP, et al. Predictors of progression from impaired glucose tolerance to NIDDM: an analysis of six prospective studies. Diabetes 1997;46:701–10.
16. Gabir MM, Hanson RL, Dabelea D, et al. The 1997 American Diabetes Association and 1999 World Health Organization criteria for hyperglycemia in the diagnosis and prediction of diabetes. Diabetes Care 2000;23:1108–12.
17. Forouhi NG, Balkau B, Borch-Johnsen K, et al. The threshold for diagnosing impaired fasting glucose: a position statement by the European Diabetes Epidemiology Group. Diabetologia 2006;49:822–7.

18. Balkau B, Hillier T, Vierron E, et al. Comment to: Borch-Johnsen K, Colagiuri S, Balkau B, et al (2004). Creating a pandemic of prediabetes: the proposed new diagnostic criteria for impaired fasting glycaemia. Diabetologia 47:1396–1402. Diabetologia 2004;47:1396–402.

19. Soderberg S, Zimmet P, Tuomilehto J, et al. High incidence of type 2 diabetes and increasing conversion rates from impaired fasting glucose and impaired glucose tolerance to diabetes in Mauritius. J Intern Med 2004;256:37–47.

20. Levitan EB, Song Y, Ford ES, et al. Is nondiabetic hyperglycemia a risk factor for cardiovascular disease? A meta-analysis of prospective studies. JAMA 2005; 293:194–202.

21. Brunner EJ, Shipley MJ, Witte DR, et al. Relation between blood glucose and coronary mortality over 33 years in the Whitehall Study. Diabetes Care 2006;29: 26–31.

22. Balkau B, Bertrais S, Ducimetiere P, et al. Is there a glycemic threshold for mortality risk? Diabetes Care 1999;22:696–9.

23. DECODE Study Group. Is the current definition for diabetes relevant to mortality risk from all causes and cardiovascular and non-cardiovascular diseases? Diabetes Care 2003;26:688–96.

24. International Expert Committee. International Expert Committee report on the role of the A1C assay in the diagnosis of diabetes. Diabetes Care 2009;32:1327–34.

25. American Diabetes Association Clinical Practice Recommendations 2010. Diabetes Care 2010;33(Suppl 1):S62–9.

26. Cowie C, Rust K, Byrd-Holt D, et al. Prevalence of diabetes and high risk for diabetes using A1C criteria in the U.S. population in 1988–2006. Diabetes Care 2010;33:562–8.

27. Ziemer DC, Kolm P, Weintraub WS, et al. Glucose-independent, black–white differences in hemoglobin A1c levels. A cross-sectional analysis of 2 studies. Ann Intern Med 2010;152:770–7.

28. Mann DM, Carson AP, Shimbo D, et al. Impact of A1C screening criterion on the diagnosis of prediabetes among U.S. adults. Diabetes Care 2010;33:2190–5.

29. Pradhan AD, Rifai N, Buring JE, et al. Hemoglobin A1c predicts diabetes but not cardiovascular disease in nondiabetic women. Am J Med 2007;120(8):720–7.

30. Selvin E, Steffes MW, Zhu H, et al. Glycated hemoglobin, diabetes, and cardiovascular risk in nondiabetic adults. N Engl J Med 2010;362:800–11.

31. Lindstrom J, Tuomilehto J. The diabetes risk score: a practical tool to predict type 2 diabetes risk. Diabetes Care 2003;26:725–31.

32. Aekplakorn W, Bunnag P, Woodward M, et al. A risk score for predicting incident diabetes in the Thai population. Diabetes Care 2006;29:1872–7.

33. Chen L, Magliano DJ, Balkau B, et al. AUSDRISK: an Australian Type 2 diabetes risk assessment tool based on demographic, lifestyle and simple anthropometric measures. Med J Aust 2010;192:197–202.

34. Hippisley-Cox J, Coupland C, Robson J, et al. Predicting risk of type 2 diabetes in England and Wales: prospective derivation and validation of QDScore. BMJ 2009;338:b880.

35. Schmidt MI, Duncan BB, Bang H, et al. Identifying individuals at high risk for diabetes: the atherosclerosis risk in communities study. Diabetes Care 2005;28: 2013–8.

36. Schulze MB, Hoffmann K, Boeing H, et al. An accurate risk score based on anthropometric, dietary, and lifestyle factors to predict the development of type 2 diabetes. Diabetes Care 2007;30:510–5.

37. Stern MP, Williams K, Haffner SM. Identification of persons at high risk for type 2 diabetes mellitus: do we need the oral glucose tolerance test? Ann Intern Med 2002;136:575–81.
38. Saaristo T, Peltonen M, Lindstrom J, et al. Cross-sectional evaluation of the Finnish Diabetes Risk Score: a tool to identify undetected type 2 diabetes, abnormal glucose tolerance and metabolic syndrome. Diab Vasc Dis Res 2005;2:67–72.

Mechanisms of Vascular Complications in Prediabetes

Sofiya Milman, MD[a], Jill P. Crandall, MD[b],*

KEYWORDS

- Prediabetes • Cardiovascular disease
- Microvascular complications • Mechanisms

Although the state of prediabetes is defined by its role as a diabetes risk factor, it also carries significant risk of cardiovascular disease (CVD). Numerous reports have documented that CVD risk is increased in prediabetes (impaired glucose tolerance [IGT] and impaired fasting glucose [IFG]) by 10% to 40% compared with populations with normal glucose regulation.[1,2] In many studies, this enhanced CVD risk remains significant even after controlling for other known risk factors, suggesting that hyperglycemia per se (even at less than the threshold for diabetes) plays an important role. However, the dysglycemia of type 2 diabetes typically exists in the context of other metabolic abnormalities, including obesity, dyslipidemia, and hypertension, leading some to propose that the increased CVD risk in individuals with prediabetes may be largely driven by the coexistence of other metabolic syndrome components.[3] Furthermore, interventions focused on lowering glycemia in patients with established diabetes have been inconsistent, showing, at most, modest CVD benefit.[4–6] Studies in prediabetes have yielded similar mixed results.[7,8] This contrasts with the evidence from type 1 diabetes studies, in particular the Diabetes Control and Complications Trial (DCCT) and Epidemiology of Diabetes Interventions and Complications (EDIC) studies, which showed a clear cardiovascular benefit of intensive glycemic control that was most evident after prolonged follow-up.[9] Prediabetes is also associated with a small, but appreciable, incidence of typical diabetic microvascular complications, including

Disclosures: Neither author has any financial disclosures or conflict of interest related to this manuscript.

[a] Division of Endocrinology, Montefiore Medical Center, Albert Einstein College of Medicine, 111 East 210 Street, Bronx, NY 10467, USA

[b] Diabetes Clinical Trials Unit, Diabetes Research and Training Center, Division of Endocrinology/Belfer 701, Albert Einstein College of Medicine, 1300 Morris Park Avenue, Bronx, NY 10461, USA

* Corresponding author.

E-mail address: jill.crandall@einstein.yu.edu

Med Clin N Am 95 (2011) 309–325

doi:10.1016/j.mcna.2010.11.004

0025-7125/11/$ – see front matter © 2011 Elsevier Inc. All rights reserved.

retinopathy, nephropathy, and neuropathy. The pathogenesis of the microvascular complications of diabetes seem to be more clearly related to duration and severity of hyperglycemia, although recent evidence suggests that other metabolic factors may contribute as well. This article reviews some of the proposed mechanisms (both glucose mediated and non–glucose mediated) for the vascular complications of the prediabetic state.

MACROVASCULAR DISEASE IN PREDIABETES
IFG Versus IGT

The state of prediabetes is heterogeneous with respect to the nature of the metabolic defect, the pattern of hyperglycemia, and the cardiovascular risk. Postchallenge hyperglycemia, including IGT, is characterized by greater skeletal muscle (peripheral) insulin resistance and compensatory hyperinsulinemia than IFG, which is associated with hepatic insulin resistance and excessive endogenous glucose production.[10] The cardiometabolic risk factors, including increased body mass index (BMI), blood pressure, and triglycerides, which often coexist in subjects with IGT and IFG, have been shown in some studies to be more pronounced in IGT.[11,12] Individuals with combined IGT and IFG seem to have a more severe metabolic defect, higher risk of progression to diabetes and a more adverse CVD risk profile.[12]

Evidence from prospective studies suggests that CVD events may be more strongly associated with IGT than IFG.[13–15] The risk for CVD and coronary heart disease (CHD) events seems to be linear, with rising postchallenge glucose levels, with a hazard ratio of 1.2 for every 1 to 2 mmol/L increase in glucose above the normal range.[13,16] In a large meta-analysis of 10 European studies, involving more than 22,000 subjects, the risk for CVD mortality was ~30% higher in those with IGT compared with the normal glucose tolerance (NGT) and IFG groups.[17] In contrast, an increased risk for cerebrovascular disease (stroke) seems to be associated with both IFG and IGT, although the strength of this relationship is not as robust as for coronary heart disease.[18,19]

Pathogenesis of Macrovascular Complications

Haffner and colleagues[20] proposed that the increased CVD risk associated with type 2 diabetes begins well before diagnostic glucose thresholds are reached (the causes of future CVD events begin to develop even in the prediabetic state).[21] Much attention has been focused on the metabolic syndrome (and its various components) as the major factor responsible for CVD risk in prediabetes, with further acceleration of risk with progression to frank diabetes (**Fig. 1**).[22] However, the contribution of episodic or mild hyperglycemia to CVD risk in the prediabetic state seems to be less certain and is the subject of active research. In addition, there is controversy as to whether the increased CVD risk associated with prediabetes can be explained by the subsequent development of overt diabetes.[23,24]

Mechanisms of Vasculopathy not Mediated by Hyperglycemia Per Se

Insulin resistance/hyperinsulinemia
Insulin resistance is characteristic of prediabetes (especially IGT) and is central to the concept of the insulin resistance syndrome as a CVD risk factor. Insulin resistance has consistently been reported to be an independent CVD risk factor in epidemiologic studies[25] and several recent clinical trials have explored the hypothesis that pharmacologic improvement of insulin sensitivity will reduce clinical CVD events.[26–28] Although these trials have failed to confirm this hypothesis, there remains strong

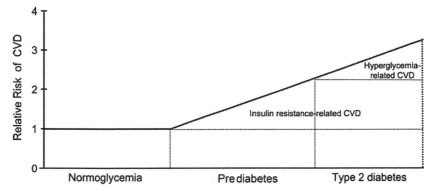

Fig. 1. Relative risk of CVD in normoglycemia, prediabetes and type 2 diabetes. (*Reprinted from* Laakso M. Cardiovascular disease in type 2 diabetes from population to man to mechanisms. Diabetes Care 2010;33:444. Copyright 2010 American Diabetes Association; with permission.)

evidence that insulin resistance does play a significant role in the development of atherosclerosis.

In vascular endothelium, the phosphatidylinositol 3-kinase (PI 3-kinase)–dependent insulin signaling pathway regulates the production of nitric oxide (NO) via stimulation of endothelial nitric oxide synthase (eNOS) activity. NO has multiple roles in vascular physiology, including vasodilation, regulation of vascular smooth muscle proliferation, and expression of cellular adhesion molecules (eg, vascular cell adhesion molecule 1 [VCAM-1], e-selectin) that are involved in initiation of atherosclerotic plaque formation.[29] NO also acts locally to inhibit platelet aggregation. Signaling via the PI 3-kinase pathway is impaired in states of insulin resistance in all insulin sensitive tissues, including endothelial cells, thus leading to reduced production of NO and attenuation of its beneficial vascular effects (**Fig. 2**). Signaling via the mitogen-activated protein kinase (MAP-kinase) pathway mediates the growth-promoting effects of insulin and remains intact in insulin-resistant states. In the setting of resistance in the PI 3-kinase pathway, there is compensatory hyperinsulinemia, and thus promotion of mitogenesis (cell proliferation) and vasoconstriction, factors that promote atherosclerosis.[30,31] In an experimental model, mice lacking endothelial insulin receptors showed impaired vasodilation, increased adhesion molecule expression, and accelerated atherosclerosis, suggesting that increased activation of the MAP-kinase pathway may not be necessary for insulin resistance to promote vascular dysfunction.[32] Thus, the normal effects of insulin to promote vascular health become distorted in the setting of insulin resistance and hyperinsulinemia.

In addition to its affects on the endothelium, insulin resistance may also have direct effects on the myocardium. In normal conditions, energy for myocardial contraction is obtained from oxidation of free fatty acids (in the fasting state) or glucose (in the fed state). In the setting of myocardial ischemia, glucose seems to be the preferred substrate, but impaired insulin-mediated glucose transport into myocytes has been proposed as a mechanism contributing to the occurrence of cardiac events and poor outcomes in insulin-resistant individuals.[33] Alterations in insulin-mediated changes in myocardial blood flow may also predispose to ischemic events.[34]

Endothelial dysfunction

Endothelial dysfunction is widely considered to be a key initiating factor in the development of atherosclerosis.[35] Impaired endothelial function caused by reduced

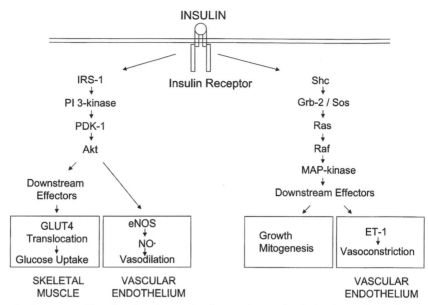

Fig. 2. Features of insulin signal transduction pathways in skeletal muscle and vascular tissue. (*Reprinted from* Kim J, Montagnani M, Koh KK, et al. Reciprocal relationships between insulin resistance and endothelial dysfunction. Circulation 2006;113:1889; with permission from Wolters Kluwer Health.)

availability of NO can be considered a manifestation of insulin resistance, as described earlier. There is also evidence that dyslipidemia, including the increased levels of free fatty acids characteristic of obesity and prediabetes, may further reduce NO availability via generation of reactive oxygen species (ROS), which act to quench NO.[36] In addition, free fatty acids and adipose-derived cytokines can inhibit the PI 3-kinase insulin signaling pathway, leading to reduced eNOS activity and NO production.[37] Hyperglycemia, even if mild and episodic, has been associated with further impairment in endothelial function, as discussed later. NO-dependent increases in blood flow to skeletal muscle may account for 25% to 40% of the glucose uptake in response to insulin stimulation, suggesting that endothelial dysfunction may contribute to insulin resistance.[37]

Obesity and inflammation
In the past decade, there has been increasing recognition of adipose tissue as an active endocrine organ that secretes a large number of cytokines and bioactive mediators that play a role in insulin sensitivity, inflammation, coagulation, and, ultimately, atherosclerosis.[38] Increased body weight may also induce morphologic and hemodynamic cardiac adaptations that increase the occurrence of clinical cardiac disease.[39]

Visceral versus subcutaneous adipose tissue Body fat distribution seems to be an important determinant of the cardiovascular risk associated with obesity.[40] The association of visceral fat with cardiometabolic risk has been shown in epidemiologic studies showing correlation of waist circumference (or waist/hip ratio) with other CVD risk factors and measures of subclinical atherosclerosis, including carotid wall thickness and arterial stiffness.[41–43] Prospective studies have shown that abdominal obesity is an independent predictor of mortality.[44] In addition, surgical removal of visceral, but not subcutaneous, fat has resulted in improvements in insulin sensitivity, lipoproteins, and blood pressure.[45–47] Visceral adipose tissue is a greater source of proinflammatory cytokines than other fat depots, which likely explains these relationships.

Inflammatory cytokines/adipokines Adipose tissue is a rich source of proinflammatory mediators that may directly contribute to vascular injury and atherosclerosis. These mediators include leptin, TNF-α, interleukin (IL)-6, resistin, and many others. Adipose tissue is also the source for the protein adiponectin, which has antiinflammatory and insulin-sensitizing properties. Recent studies have revealed the importance of adipose tissue macrophages as a significant source of inflammatory signals in obesity. The density of adipose macrophages is increased in obesity, particularly in visceral fat depots, providing further evidence of obesity as a proinflammatory state.[48,49]

Leptin The adipokine leptin is best known for its role in regulation of body weight and energy expenditure. However, functional leptin receptors have been identified in vascular tissues including endothelial cells, vascular smooth muscle cells, and platelets. The hyperleptinemia characteristic of human obesity has been linked to endothelial dysfunction and activation of the sympathetic nervous system.[50] Leptin also has proinflammatory properties and can stimulate the proliferation of smooth muscle cells, which plays a role in growth of atherosclerotic plaque.[51,52] Leptin has been shown to promote platelet aggregation and arterial thrombosis in some animal models, although its role in human thrombotic disorders is not clear.[53]

TNF-α TNF-α plays a key role in atherosclerosis via its activation of the transcription factor nuclear factor-κB (NF-κB). This results in expression of adhesion molecules (eg, VCAM-1, interstitial cell adhesion molecule 1, e-selectin, and monocyte chemoattractive protein-1 [MCP-1]) that promote attachment of circulating monocytes and their migration into the vessel wall, thus initiating foam cell formation. TNF-α may also impair endothelial function by reducing availability of NO and has been shown to promote endothelial cell apoptosis.[54,55]

IL-6 and C-reactive protein IL-6 is secreted by a variety of immune cells (eg, T cells, monocytes), but up to one-third of circulating IL-6 is derived from adipose tissue.[56] IL-6 regulates hepatic production of C-reactive protein (CRP), which has emerged as an important inflammatory marker that is increased in direct proportion to body fat mass. CRP also seems to have a direct cellular action of its own. CRP induces endothelial cell expression of adhesion molecules, reduces the availability of NO, and may play a coordinating role by amplifying the proinflammatory activity of other cytokines.[57]

Adiponectin Adiponectin is abundantly expressed in adipocytes but, unlike other adipokines, circulating levels are reduced in obesity. Adiponectin has important insulin-sensitizing and antiatherosclerotic properties. It has favorable effects on endothelial function, including stimulation of nitric oxide production and reduction in expression of cellular adhesion molecules via effects on the transcription factor, NF-κB.[58,59] Adiponectin has other antiinflammatory properties and there is evidence that it may protect from atherosclerotic plaque rupture via inhibition of matrix metalloproteinase function.[60]

Atherogenic dyslipidemia
The characteristic diabetic dyslipidemia with increased triglycerides, low high-density lipoprotein (HDL) cholesterol and small, dense low-density lipoprotein (LDL) particles,

is also present in insulin-resistant, prediabetic individuals. This lipid profile is a central component of the metabolic syndrome, which defines a state of increased CVD risk. A detailed discussion of lipid physiology in insulin resistance/prediabetes has been the subject of several recent reviews.[61,62] Overproduction of large triglyceride-rich very-low-density lipoprotein (VLDL) particles, which may occur as a consequence of insulin resistance, is emerging as a key factor leading to an atherogenic lipid profile. This overproduction of VLDL particles leads to further lipid permutations, resulting in high levels of remnant particles, small dense LDL and low levels of HDL-cholesterol. These small dense LDL particles are more prone to oxidation and more readily enter the vessel wall, initiating the process of atherosclerotic plaque formation.

Thrombosis and fibrinolysis

Established type 2 diabetes is known to constitute a prothrombotic state, caused by abnormalities in platelet function, coagulation factors, and fibrinolysis.[63,64] There is also substantial evidence for prothrombosis in prediabetes and the metabolic syndrome.[65] The most consistent finding has been increased levels of plasminogen activator inhibitor-1 (PAI-1), which results in impaired fibrinolysis, thus tipping the balance in favor of thrombosis. PAI-1 levels are closely associated with obesity and insulin resistance, and both baseline levels and increases with time were shown to predict the development of type 2 diabetes.[66,67] Circulating PAI-1 is derived primarily from adipose tissue, particularly stromal cells and macrophages. Increased levels of factor VII, abnormal platelet function (caused by decreased availability of NO), and increased levels of fibrinogen have also been described in obesity and insulin resistance.[68,69]

Mechanisms of Vasculopathy Linked to Hyperglycemia Per Se

The processes by which hyperglycemia per se contributes to vascular damage are multiple and complex. Studies in vitro have shown that high glucose exposure results in activation of the proinflammatory transcription factor, NF-κB, production of advanced glycation end products, generation of ROS, enhanced monocyte adhesion to endothelial cells, and inhibition of NO production.[70] Increased ROS generation further leads to oxidation of LDL, rendering it significantly more atherogenic. Hyperglycemia also seems to induce a prothrombotic state by inducing platelet activation and increasing the synthesis of PAI-1. Although many different pathways seem to be involved in mediating the vascular effects of high glucose, a unifying theory of the biochemical basis of hyperglycemic cellular damage, which implicates overproduction of superoxide by the mitochondrial electron transport chain, has been proposed as the key process.[71] In most cases, these pathologic mechanisms have been shown in conditions of prolonged exposure to extreme glucose increases, but they also have relevance to vascular dysfunction in prediabetic states that are characterized by mild and/or transient hyperglycemia. This article focuses on mechanisms with particular or unique relevance to transient or episodic mild hyperglycemia.

Postchallenge hyperglycemia

Postchallenge (following an oral glucose load) or postprandial (following a meal) hyperglycemia is characteristic of prediabetes and has been associated with increased CVD risk in observational studies.[17] Postchallenge hyperglycemia (ie, IGT) has consistently been reported to be a better predictor of CVD and total mortality than fasting glucose levels and is correlated with the presence of subclinical atherosclerosis and other CVD markers.[72,73] Following a typical high-carbohydrate meal, individuals with IGT are exposed to higher peak and sustained levels of glucose, indicating that repeated postmeal glucose spikes are a frequent, but unrecognized, occurrence in this population.[74] These brief periods of hyperglycemia have been reported to induce vascular dysfunction, providing a mechanistic link between episodic glucose increases and CVD risk. Postchallenge hyperglycemia is largely an age-related phenomenon, occurring in up to 30% of people more than 60 years of age.[75] Older adults with IGT have higher levels of CRP, lower levels of adiponectin, and an overall adverse CVD risk profile compared with age- and BMI-matched control subjects with normal glucose regulation.[74]

Oxidative stress

Substantial attention has been focused on oxidative stress as a central mechanism explaining the increased CVD risk associated with acute, episodic hyperglycemia, although the issue remains confounded by lack of consensus on appropriate methodology for quantifying ROS in vivo.[76] In vitro studies have shown increased production of ROS in cultured endothelial and vascular smooth muscle cells exposed to brief periods of high glucose.[77] In vivo studies have also reported reduction of plasma antioxidants following an oral glucose load and increased levels of nitrotyrosine (an oxidative stress marker) with short-term (120 minutes) exposure to hyperglycemia in healthy subjects.[78] Urinary excretion of F2-isoprostanes (another oxidative stress marker) showed stronger correlation with acute glucose fluctuations and postprandial glucose area under the curve than with mean glucose levels in a study of type 2 diabetes patients using continuous glucose monitoring.[79]

Endothelial dysfunction

Endothelial dysfunction has frequently been reported with both chronic and acute hyperglycemia and may be mediated by generation of ROS and consequent inactivation of NO.[80,81] Impaired endothelium-dependent vasodilation has been reported in subjects with IGT following an oral sugar load or a high-carbohydrate meal and shows inverse correlation with plasma glucose levels in some studies.[74,82–84] Similar effects have been inconsistently reported in subjects with NGT, with evidence to suggest that the less-pronounced glycemic excursion in control subjects may be insufficient to induce vascular dysfunction.[85,86] In addition, insulin-induced vasodilation remains intact in individuals with normal insulin sensitivity and may temper the effects of hyperglycemia. Postchallenge endothelial dysfunction has been correlated with oxidative stress markers and restored with administration of antioxidants (vitamins and α lipoic acid), thus implicating glucose-induced ROS generation as a likely mechanism.[83,85,87,88] Reversal of impaired endothelial function with lowering of postchallenge hyperglycemia, using the nonabsorbable drug acarbose, has been reported and provides further evidence to implicate hyperglycemia per se in this phenomenon.[82]

Inflammation and thrombosis

Acute hyperglycemia, either sustained for 5 hours or in 2-hour pulses has resulted in increases of circulating levels of inflammatory cytokines, including IL-6, IL-18 and TNF-α, with more pronounced effects observed in subjects with IGT compared with NGT.[89] These effects were abolished by coadministration of the antioxidant glutathione, again implicating oxidative stress as a mechanism. Alteration in several hemostatic factors have been reported in subjects with IGT, including increased levels of PAI-1, von Willebrand factor, and tissue plasminogen activator, and show correlation with fasting and 2-hour glucose.[90] Short-term (6 hour) hyperglycemia in nondiabetic control subjects induced a procoagulant effect, which was exacerbated by combined hyperglycemia and hyperinsulinemia, although the relevance of this observation to shorter hyperglycemic episodes (ie, postprandial) is unclear.[91] In a study of early type 2 diabetes with mild hyperglycemia, lowering of postprandial glucose with the drug acarbose resulted in reduction in platelet activation, again suggesting a role for transient glucose spikes in the promotion of a prothrombotic state.[92]

Epigenetic modification

Recent interest in the role of glycemic variability in the pathogenesis of vasculopathy, as well as the phenomenon of metabolic memory, has led to exploration of potential molecular mechanisms. Transient exposure of aortic endothelial cells to hyperglycemia induced long-lasting epigenetic changes in the promoter of the NF-κB gene, which resulted in increased expression of inflammatory genes in vitro.[93] This effect was confirmed in an animal model and persisted for several days after normalization of glucose, highlighting the potential contribution of even short-term hyperglycemia to persistent vascular damage.

MICROVASCULAR COMPLICATIONS IN PREDIABETES

In the past few decades, glucose thresholds for the diagnosis of diabetes have been debated and revised, but the foundation for selection of a diabetes cutoff point is the glucose level at which typical diabetic microvascular complications begin to emerge. However, it has also been appreciated that glucose levels exist on a continuum and that diabetic retinopathy, nephropathy, and neuropathy do occur at lower levels among individuals with prediabetes or even normoglycemia. Although these microvascular changes may be mild, they are clinically significant in some cases and can provide insight into the mechanisms and natural history of diabetic vasculopathy. In general, microvascular complications seen in prediabetes have been attributed solely to hyperglycemia. However, recent evidence supports a potential pathogenic role for other metabolic factors, including obesity, dyslipidemia, and hypertension. Further evidence comes from a study suggesting that the metabolic syndrome has an additive effect on the risk of microvascular complications in patients with established diabetes.[94]

Nephropathy

Impaired glucose regulation is associated with albuminuria and renal dysfunction. The National Health and Nutrition Examination Survey (NHANES) data from 1999 to 2006 revealed that the prevalence of chronic kidney disease (urinary albumin/creatinine ratio of >30 mg/g or eGFR <60 mL/min per 1.73 m^2) was 17% in those with IFG compared with 12% in those with NGT.[95] There seems to be a threshold effect for this phenomenon, with a doubling in prevalent albuminuria (to 20%) at a HbA1c level of 6.1%.[96] Microalbuminuric subjects with IGT or IFG have significantly higher eGFR compared with those with NGT, suggesting that the hyperfiltration associated with early diabetic nephropathy exists even in the prediabetic state.[97] Albuminuria is also a predictor of CVD events and mortality, even in the absence of progression to clinical nephropathy.[98,99]

Nonglycemic risk factors may contribute to renal disease in prediabetic individuals. Studies in varied ethnic populations have documented independent associations of albuminuria with obesity, hypertension, and dyslipidemia.[100,101] Obesity has a particularly strong association with chronic kidney disease, with increases in inflammatory fat-derived peptides (eg, leptin, IL-6, TNF-α) and low levels of adiponectin proposed as potential mechanisms. Increased leptin levels may lead to proliferation of glomerular endothelial cells and increased synthesis of type VI collagen, resulting in glomerulosclerosis and proteinuria.[102] Leptin may also contribute to renal dysfunction via an increase in sympathetic tone, sodium retention, and resulting hypertension.[102] The hypoadiponectinemia of obesity may cause a reduction in activity of 5'-AMP activated protein kinase (AMPK), which has antiproliferative effects on mesangial cells, and ultimately results in mesangial expansion and proteinuria.[103] The dyslipidemia associated with insulin resistance seems to be a significant contributor to nephropathy. Increased circulating levels of free fatty acids promote the formation of ROS and can lead to renal cell injury.[104] High levels of triglyceride-rich lipoproteins may promote mesangial proliferation, a typical feature of diabetic nephropathy.[102]

Retinopathy

The prevalence of typical early diabetic retinopathy in populations with prediabetes has been reported to be as high as 8%, with higher rates observed with more severe hyperglycemia (combined IFG and IGT).[105–108] However, the clinical significance of retinopathy in prediabetes is uncertain, because it is described in most studies as very mild, often a single microaneurysm or hemorrhage that may regress during follow-up.[109] Studies of retinopathy in subjects with prediabetes are confounded by the association of retinopathy with hypertension and obesity.[110,111] Hypertensive retinopathy has many overlapping features with diabetic retinopathy, at times making the distinction difficult.[112] There is little evidence whether other nonglycemic factors (eg, dyslipidemia) make a significant contribution to retinopathy in prediabetes.

Neuropathy

Peripheral and autonomic neuropathies have been found in association with prediabetes, with the prevalence appearing to be higher in prediabetes (13% and 11.3% in IGT and IFG, respectively), compared with age-matched NGT subjects (7.4%).[113] However, the precise prevalence is difficult to estimate in part because the neuropathy caused by diabetes is not distinct in its symptoms or examination findings from neuropathies from other causes. Neuropathy occurring in prediabetes generally affects small unmyelinated or lightly myelinated axons that transmit pain and autonomic signals.[114] The most common symptoms of peripheral neuropathy reported by subjects with prediabetes are sensory complaints and do not differ from those with typical diabetic neuropathy.[115] However, the neuropathy associated with IGT is less severe than the neuropathy seen with diabetes, documented by skin nerve fiber density, nerve amplitude, and nerve velocity.[116] Manifestations of autonomic neuropathy have also been found in association with prediabetes, mostly attributed to vagal dysautonomia.[117,118] Middle-aged subjects with IFG manifest a decrease in heart rate recovery after exercise testing, a marker of reduced parasympathetic activity, compared with age-matched NGT controls. In addition, abnormal heart rate recovery added to IFG for the prediction of mortality in this study.[117] Other manifestations of autonomic dysfunction noted in IGT include diminished heart rate variation and impaired postural changes in blood pressure and heart rate.[118]

Waist circumference, dyslipidemia, increased blood pressure, and age have emerged as risk factors for polyneuropathy in prediabetic subjects.[113,118–120] Dysfunction of small nerve fibers was found in subjects with metabolic syndrome and IGT; these neuronal changes were not seen in healthy controls or subjects with type 1 diabetes, suggesting that metabolic syndrome, not glycemic burden, was the contributing factor.[121] Supporting evidence for this association comes from a study of patients with established diabetes, in whom those with the metabolic syndrome were twice as likely to have polyneuropathy compared with those without the

---

Box 1
Mechanisms proposed for macro- and microvascular dysfunction in prediabetes

Non–glucose mediated

Insulin resistance and/or hyperinsulinemia

    Reduced NO synthesis→endothelial dysfunction

    Impaired glucose uptake in cardiac myocytes

    Altered insulin-mediated myocardial blood flow

Obesity and inflammation

    Adipocytokines

    Oxidative stress

Dyslipidemia

    Atherogenic lipoproteins

    Increased circulating free fatty acids→ROS generation

Prothrombosis

    Increased levels of PAI-1

    Platelet activation

Glucose mediated (transient or episodic hyperglycemia)

Oxidative stress

    Inactivation of NO→endothelial dysfunction,

    Increased inflammatory cytokine expression

    Oxidation of lipoproteins

Prothrombosis

    Increased levels of PAI-1

    Increased levels of coagulation factors

    Enhanced platelet activation

Epigenetic modification

    Increased expression of inflammatory genes via NF-κB

---

metabolic syndrome.[122] Obesity-induced oxidative stress has also been implicated in the pathogenesis of polyneuropathy.[123]

SUMMARY

The occurrence of typical diabetic macro- and microvascular complications in the prediabetic state emphasizes the continuous nature of the relationship between glycemia and vascular health. The additional contribution of other metabolic factors is apparent from the wealth of recent research and highlights the complexity of the pathologic processes involved. The failure of glucose-centered interventions to meaningfully reduce macrovascular disease in established diabetes presents a challenge to both the clinical care of patients with diabetes and prediabetes, as well as to our understanding of key disease mechanisms. Additional research is needed to clarify the role of glucose- and non–glucose-mediated processes, which will hopefully lead to improved therapeutic strategies (**Box 1**).

REFERENCES

1. Levitsky Y, Pencina M, D'Agostino R, et al. Impact of impaired fasting glucose on cardiovascular disease. J Am Coll Cardiol 2008;51:264–70.
2. Coutinho M, Gerstein HC, Wang Y, et al. The relationship between glucose and incident cardiovascular events. A meta-regression analysis of published data from 20 studies of 95,783 individuals followed for 12.4 years. Diabetes Care 1999;22:233–40.
3. Liu J, Grundy S, Wang W, et al. Ten-year risk of cardiovascular incidence related to diabetes, prediabetes and the metabolic syndrome. Am Heart J 2007;153: 552–8.
4. The Action to Control Cardiovascular Risk in Diabetes Study Group. Effects of intensive glucose lowering in type 2 diabetes. N Engl J Med 2008;358: 2545–59.
5. Patel A, MacMahon S, Chalmers J, et al, The ADVANCE Collaborative Group. ADVANCE: intensive blood glucose control and vascular outcomes in patients with type 2 diabetes. N Engl J Med 2008;358:2560–72.
6. Holman R, Paul SK, Bethel MA, et al. UKPDS 10-year follow-up of intensive glucose control in type 2 diabetes. N Engl J Med 2008;359:1577–89.
7. The NAVIGATOR Study Group. Effect of nateglinide on the incidence of diabetes and cardiovascular events. N Engl J Med 2010;362:1463–76.
8. Chiasson JL, Josse RG, Gomis R, et al. Acarbose treatment and the risk of cardiovascular disease and hypertension in patients with impaired glucose tolerance: the STOP-NIDDM trial. JAMA 2003;290:486–94.
9. Nathan DM, Cleary PA, Backlund JY, et al. Intensive diabetes treatment and cardiovascular disease in patients with type 1 diabetes. N Engl J Med 2005; 353:2643–53.
10. Abdul-Ghani MA, Tripathy D, DeFronzo R. Contributions of beta cell dysfunction and insulin resistance to the pathogenesis of impaired glucose tolerance and impaired fasting glucose. Diabetes Care 2006;29:1130–9.
11. Haffner SM, Mykkanen L, Festa A, et al. Insulin-resistant prediabetic subjects have more atherogenic risk factors than insulin sensitive prediabetic subjects: implications for preventing coronary heart disease during the prediabetic state. Circulation 2000;101:975–80.
12. Pankow JS, Kwan DK, Duncan BB, et al. Cardiometabolic risk in impaired fasting glucose and impaired glucose tolerance. The Atherosclerosis Risk in Communities study. Diabetes Care 2007;30:325–31.
13. Brunner EJ, Shipley MJ, Witte DR, et al. Relationship between blood glucose and coronary mortality over 33 years in the Whitehall Study. Diabetes Care 2006;29:26–31.
14. Meigs JB, Nathan DM, D'Agostino RB, et al. Fasting and post challenge glycemia and cardiovascular disease risk. Framingham Offspring Study. Diabetes Care 2002;25:1845–50.
15. Blake DR, Meigs JB, Muller DC, et al. Impaired glucose tolerance, but not impaired fasting glucose, is associated with increased levels of coronary heart disease risk factors. Results from the Baltimore Longitudinal Study on Aging. Diabetes 2004;53:2095–100.
16. Barr ELM, Boyko EJ, Zimmet PZ, et al. Continuous relationship between non-diabetic hyperglycemia and both cardiovascular disease and all cause mortality: the Australian Diabetes, Obesity, and Lifestyle (AusDiab) Study. Diabetologia 2009;52:415–24.

17. DECODE Study Group. Glucose tolerance and cardiovascular mortality. Arch Intern Med 2001;161:397–404.

18. Tanne D, Koren-Morag N, Goldbourt U. Fasting plasma glucose and risk of incident ischemic stroke or transient ischemic attack. Stroke 2004;35:2351–5.

19. Selvin E, Steffes MW, Zhu H, et al. Glycated hemoglobin, diabetes, and cardiovascular risk in nondiabetic adults. N Engl J Med 2010;362:800–11.

20. Haffner S, Stern M, Hazuda H, et al. Cardiovascular risk factors in confirmed prediabetic individuals. JAMA 1990;263:2893–8.

21. Hu F, Stampfer M, Haffner S, et al. Elevated risk of cardiovascular disease prior to clinical diagnosis of type 2 diabetes. Diabetes Care 2002;25:1129–34.

22. Laakso M. Cardiovascular disease in type 2 diabetes from population to man to mechanisms. Diabetes Care 2010;33:442–9.

23. Qiao Q, Jousilahti P, Eriksson J, et al. Predictive properties of impaired glucose tolerance for cardiovascular risk are not explained by the development of overt diabetes during follow-up. Diabetes Care 2003;26:2910–4.

24. Rijkeljkhuizen J, Nijpels G, Heine R, et al. High risk of cardiovascular mortality in individuals with impaired fasting glucose is explained by conversion to diabetes. Diabetes Care 2007;30:332–6.

25. Rutter M, Meigs J, Sullivan L, et al. Insulin resistance, the metabolic syndrome and incident cardiovascular events in the Framingham Offspring Study. Diabetes 2005;54:3252–7.

26. Dormandy JA, Charbonnel B, Eckland DJA, et al. Secondary prevention of macrovascular events in patients with type 2 diabetes in the PROACTIVE study: a randomised controlled trial. Lancet 2005;366:1279–89.

27. The BARI 2D Study Group. BARI-2D: a randomized trial of therapies for type 2 diabetes and coronary artery disease. N Engl J Med 2009;360:2503–15.

28. Home P, Pocock SJ, Beck-Nielsen H, et al. Rosiglitazone evaluated for cardiovascular outcomes in oral agent combination therapy for type 2 diabetes (RECORD): a multicentre, randomised, open label trial. Lancet 2009;373: 2125–35.

29. Bian K, Doursout M, Murad F. Vascular system: role of nitric oxide in cardiovascular diseases. J Clin Hypertens (Greenwich) 2008;10:304–10.

30. Montagnani M, Golovchenko I, Kim I, et al. Inhibition of phosphatidylinositol 3-kinase enhances mitogenic actions of insulin in endothelial cells. J Biol Chem 2002;277:1794–9.

31. Cusi K, Maezano K, Osman A, et al. Insulin resistance differentially affects the PI 3-kinase and MAP-kinase-mediated signaling in human muscle. J Clin Invest 2000;105:311–20.

32. Rask-Madsen C, Li Q, Freund B, et al. Loss of insulin signaling in vascular endothelial cells accelerates atherosclerosis in apolipoprotein E null mice. Cell Metab 2010;11:379–89.

33. Ferrannini E, Iozzo P. Is insulin resistance atherogenic? Atheroscler Suppl 2006; 7:5–10.

34. Iozzo P, Chareonthaitawee P, Rimoldi O, et al. Mismatch between insulin-mediated glucose uptake and blood flow in the heart of patients with type II diabetes. Diabetologia 2002;45:1404–9.

35. Bonetti P, Lerman L, Lerman A. Endothelial dysfunction: a marker of atherosclerotic risk. Arterioscler Thromb Vasc Biol 2003;23:168–75.

36. Tripathy D, Mohanty P, Dhindsa S, et al. Elevation of free fatty acids induces inflammation and impairs vascular reactivity in healthy subjects. Diabetes 2003;52:2882–7.

37. Kim J, Montagnani M, Koh KK, et al. Reciprocal relationships between insulin resistance and endothelial dysfunction. Circulation 2006;113:1888–904.
38. Fantuzzi G, Mazzone T. Adipose tissue and atherosclerosis: exploring the connection. Arterioscler Thromb Vasc Biol 2007;27:996–1003.
39. Poirier P, Giles T, Bray G, et al. Obesity and cardiovascular disease: pathophysiology, evaluation and effect of weight loss. Circulation 2006;113:898–918.
40. Mathieu P, Poirier P, Pibarot P, et al. Visceral obesity: the link among inflammation, hypertension and cardiovascular disease. Hypertension 2009;53:577–84.
41. Okura T, Nakata Y, Yamabuki K, et al. Regional body composition changes exhibit opposing effects on coronary heart disease risk factors. Arterioscler Thromb Vasc Biol 2004;24:923–9.
42. Ferreira I, Snijder M, Twisk JWR, et al. Central fat mass versus peripheral fat and lean mass: opposite associations with arterial stiffness? J Clin Endocrinol Metab 2004;89:2632–9.
43. DeMichele M, Panico S, Ianuzzi A, et al. Association of obesity and central fat distribution with carotid artery wall thickening in middle-aged women. Stroke 2002;33:2923–8.
44. Kuk JL, Katzmarzyk PT, Nichaman MZ, et al. Visceral fat is an independent predictor of all-cause mortality in men. Obesity (Silver Spring) 2006;14:336–42.
45. Gabriely I, Ma X, Yan GX, et al. Removal of visceral fat prevents insulin resistance and glucose intolerance of aging: an adipokine mediated process? Diabetes 2002;51:2951–8.
46. Brochu M, Tchernoff A, Turner AN, et al. Is there a threshold of visceral fat loss that improves the metabolic profile in obese postmenopausal women? Metabolism 2003;52:599–604.
47. Klein S, Fontana L, Young VL, et al. Absence of an effect of liposuction on insulin action and risk factors for coronary heart disease. N Engl J Med 2004;350:2549–57.
48. Weisberg SP, McCann D, Desai M, et al. Obesity is associated with macrophage accumulation in adipose tissue. J Clin Invest 2003;112:1796–808.
49. Cancello R, Clement K. Is obesity an inflammatory illness? Role of low-grade inflammation and macrophage infiltration in human white adipose tissue. BJOG 2006;113:1141–7.
50. Knudsen J, Payne G, Borbouse L, et al. Leptin and mechanisms of endothelial dysfunction and cardiovascular disease. Curr Hypertens Rep 2008;10:434–9.
51. Fantuzzi G, Faggioni R. Leptin in the regulation of immunity, inflammation, and hematopoiesis. J Leukoc Biol 2000;68:437–46.
52. Yang R, Barouch LA. Leptin signaling and obesity: cardiovascular consequences. Circ Res 2007;101:545–59.
53. Wannamethee SG, Tchernova J, Whincup P, et al. Plasma leptin: associations with metabolic, inflammatory and haemostatic risk factors for cardiovascular disease. Atherosclerosis 2007;191(2):418–26.
54. Wang P, Ba ZF, Chaudry IH. Administration of tumor necrosis factor alpha in vivo depresses endothelium-dependent relaxation. Am J Physiol 1994;266:H2535–41.
55. Choy JC, Granville DJ, Hunt DW, et al. Endothelial cell apoptosis: biochemical characteristics and potential implications for atherosclerosis. J Mol Cell Cardiol 2001;33:1673–90.
56. Mohamed-Ali V, Goodrick S, Rawesh A, et al. Subcutaneous adipose tissue releases interleukin-6, but not tumor necrosis factor alpha in vivo. J Clin Endocrinol Metab 1997;82:4196–200.

57. Devaraj S, Xu DY, Jialal I. C-reactive protein increases plasminogen activating inhibitor-1 expression and activity in human aortic endothelial cells: implications for the metabolic syndrome and atherothrombosis. Circulation 2003;107: 398–404.
58. Cheng KK, Lam KS, Wang Y, et al. Adiponectin-induced endothelial nitric oxide synthase activation and nitric oxide production are mediated by APPL1 in endothelial cells. Diabetes 2007;56:1387–94.
59. Ouchi N, Kihara S, Arita Y, et al. Adiponectin, an adipocyte-derived plasma protein, inhibits endothelial NF-kappaB signaling though a cAMP-dependent pathway. Circulation 2000;102:1296–301.
60. Kumada M, Kihara S, Ouchi N, et al. Adiponectin specifically increased tissue inhibitor of metalloproteinase-1 through interleukin-10 expression in human macrophages. Circulation 2004;109:2046–9.
61. Ginsberg H, Zhang YL, Hernandez-Ono A. Metabolic syndrome: focus on dyslipidemia. Obesity (Silver Spring) 2006;14:41S–9S.
62. Adiels M, Olofsson S, Taskinen M, et al. Overproduction of very low-density lipoproteins is the hallmark of dyslipidemia in the metabolic syndrome. Arterioscler Thromb Vasc Biol 2008;28:1225–36.
63. Grant PJ. Diabetes mellitus as a prothrombotic condition. J Intern Med 2007; 262:157–72.
64. Osende J, Badimon J, Fuster V, et al. Blood thrombogenicity in type 2 diabetes is associated with glycemic control. J Am Coll Cardiol 2001;38:1307–12.
65. Mansfield M, Heywood DM, Grant PJ. Circulating levels of factor VII, fibrinogen and von Willebrand factor and features of insulin resistance in first degree relatives of patients with NIDDM. Circulation 1996;94:2171–6.
66. Festa A, Williams K, Tracy R, et al. Progression of plasminogen activator-1 and fibrinogen levels in relation to incident type 2 diabetes. Circulation 2006;113: 1753–9.
67. Mertens I, Verrijkens A, Michiels JJ, et al. Among inflammation and coagulation markers, PAI-1 is a true component of the metabolic syndrome. Int J Obes (Lond) 2006;30(8):1308–14.
68. Sakkinen P, Wahl P, Cushman M, et al. Clustering of procoagulation, inflammation and fibrinolysis variables with metabolic factors in insulin resistance syndrome. Am J Epidemiol 2000;152:897–907.
69. Meigs J, Mittleman M, Nathan D, et al. Hyperinsulinemia, hyperglycemia and impaired hemostasis: the Framingham Offspring Study. JAMA 2000;283:221–8.
70. Mazzone T, Chair A, Plutzky J. Cardiovascular disease risk in type 2 diabetes: insights from mechanistic studies. Lancet 2008;371:1800–9.
71. Brownlee M. The pathobiology of diabetic complications: a unifying hypothesis. Diabetes 2005;54:1615–25.
72. Saydah SH, Miret M, Sung J, et al. Postchallenge hyperglycemia and mortality in a national sample of US adults. Diabetes Care 2001;24:1397–402.
73. Hanfeld M, Kroehler C, Henkel E, et al. Post-challenge hyperglycemia relates more strongly than fasting hyperglycemia with carotid intima-media thickness: the RIAD Study. Diabet Med 2000;17:835–40.
74. Crandall JP, Shamoon H, Cohen H, et al. Post-challenge hyperglycemia in older adults is associated with increased cardiovascular risk. J Clin Endocrinol Metab 2009;94:1595–601.
75. Centers for Disease Control and Prevention. National diabetes fact sheet: general information and national estimates on diabetes in the United States,

2007. Atlanta (GA): US Department of Health and Human Services, Centers for Disease Control and Prevention; 2008.
76. Choi SW, Bensie I, Ma SW, et al. Acute hyperglycemia and oxidative stress: direct cause and effect? Free Radic Biol Med 2008;4:1217–31.
77. Inoguchi T, Li P, Umeda F, et al. High glucose level and free fatty acid stimulate reactive oxygen species production through protein kinase C-dependent activation of NAD(P)H oxidase in cultured vascular cells. Diabetes 2000;49:1939–45.
78. Marfella R, Quagliaro L, Nappo F, et al. Acute hyperglycemia induces oxidative stress in healthy subjects. J Clin Invest 2001;108:635–6.
79. Monnier L, Mas E, Ginet C, et al. Activation of oxidative stress by acute glucose fluctuations compared with sustained chronic hyperglycemia in patients with type 2 diabetes. JAMA 2006;295:1681–7.
80. Williams SB, Goldfine AB, Timimi FK, et al. Acute hyperglycemia attenuates endothelium-dependent vasodilation in humans in vivo. Circulation 1998;97: 1695–701.
81. Johnstone MT, Creager SJ, Scales KM, et al. Impaired endothelium-dependent vasodilation in patients with insulin dependent diabetes mellitus. Circulation 1993;88:2510–6.
82. Wascher TC, Schmoelzer I, Wiegratz A, et al. Reduction in postchallenge hyperglycemia prevents acute endothelial dysfunction in subjects with impaired glucose tolerance. Eur J Clin Invest 2005;35:551–7.
83. Xiang G, Sun H, Zhao L, et al. The antioxidant alpha-lipoic acid improves endothelial dysfunction induced by acute hyperglycemia during OGTT in impaired glucose tolerance. Clin Endocrinol 2008;68:716–23.
84. Kawano H, Motoyama T, Hirashima O, et al. Hyperglycemia rapidly suppresses flow-mediated endothelium-dependent vasodilation of the brachial artery. J Am Coll Cardiol 1999;34:146–54.
85. Title L, Cummings P, Giddens K, et al. Oral glucose loading acutely attenuates endothelium-dependent vasodilation in healthy adults without diabetes: an effect prevented by vitamins C and E. J Am Coll Cardiol 2000;36:2185–91.
86. Major-Pedersen A, Ihlemann N, Hermann T, et al. Effects of oral glucose load on endothelial function and on insulin and glucose fluctuations in healthy individuals. Exp Diabetes Res 2008:672021.
87. Beckman J, Goldfine A, Gordon M, et al. Ascorbate restores endothelium-dependent vasodilation impaired by acute hyperglycemia in humans. Circulation 2001;103:1618–23.
88. Neri S, Signorelli SS, Torrisi B, et al. Effects of antioxidant supplementation on postprandial oxidative stress and endothelial dysfunction: a single-blind, 15-day clinical trial in patients with untreated type 2 diabetes, subjects with impaired glucose tolerance and healthy controls. Clin Ther 2005;27:1764–73.
89. Esposito K, Nappo F, Marfella R, et al. Inflammatory cytokine concentrations are acutely increased by hyperglycemia in humans: role of oxidative stress. Circulation 2002;106:2067–72.
90. Leurs P, Stolk R, Hamulyak K, et al. Tissue factor pathway inhibitor and other endothelium-dependent hemostatic factors in elderly individuals with normal or impaired glucose tolerance and type 2 diabetes. Diabetes Care 2002;25: 1340–5.
91. Stegenga M, van der Crabben S, Levi M, et al. Hyperglycemia stimulates coagulation, whereas hyperinsulinemia impairs fibrinolysis in healthy humans. Diabetes 2006;55:1807–12.

92. Santilli F, Formoso G, Sbraccia P, et al. Postprandial hyperglycemia is a determinant of platelet activation in early type 2 diabetes mellitus. J Thromb Haemost 2010;8:828–37.

93. El-Osta A, Brassachio D, Yao D, et al. Transient high glucose causes persistent epigenetic changes and altered gene expression during subsequent normoglycemia. J Exp Med 2008;205:2409–17.

94. Isomma B, Henricsson M, Almgren P, et al. The metabolic syndrome influences the risk of chronic complications in patients with type II diabetes. Diabetologia 2001;44:1148–54.

95. Plantinga LC, Crews DC, Coresh J, et al. Prevalence of chronic kidney disease in US adults with undiagnosed diabetes or prediabetes. Clin J Am Soc Nephrol 2010;5:673–82.

96. Tapp RJ, Zimmet PZ, Harper CA, et al. Diagnostic thresholds for diabetes: the association of retinopathy and albuminuria with glycaemia. Diabetes Res Clin Pract 2006;73:315–21.

97. Jia W, Gao X, Pang C, et al. Prevalence and risk factors of albuminuria and chronic kidney disease in Chinese population with type 2 diabetes and impaired glucose regulation: Shanghai Diabetic Complications Study (SHDCS). Nephrol Dial Transplant 2009;24:3724–31.

98. Gerstein HC, Mann JFE, Yi Q, et al. Albuminuria and risk of cardiovascular events, death, and heart failure in diabetic and nondiabetic individuals. JAMA 2001;286:421–6.

99. Hemmelgarn BR, Manns BJ, Lloyd A, et al. Relation between kidney function, proteinuria, and adverse outcomes. JAMA 2010;303:423–9.

100. Atkins RC, Polkinghorne KR, Briganti EM, et al. Prevalence of albuminuria in Australia: the AusDiab Kidney Study. Kidney Int Suppl 2004;92:S22–4.

101. Okpechi IG, Pascone MD, Swanepoel CR, et al. Microalbuminuria and the metabolic syndrome in non-diabetic black Africans. Diab Vasc Dis Res 2007; 4:365–7.

102. Wahba IM, Mak RH. Obesity and obesity-initiated metabolic syndrome: mechanistic links to chronic kidney disease. Clin J Am Soc Nephrol 2007; 2(3):550–62.

103. Ix JH, Sharma K. Mechanisms linking obesity, chronic kidney disease, and fatty liver disease: the roles of fetuin-A, adiponectin, and AMPK. J Am Soc Nephrol 2010;21:406–12.

104. Steinberg HO, Tarshoby M, Monestel R, et al. Elevated circulating free fatty acid levels impair endothelium-dependent vasodilation. J Clin Invest 1997;100:1230–9.

105. Wong TY, Barr ELM, Tapp RJ, et al. Retinopathy in persons with impaired glucose metabolism: the Australian Diabetes Obesity Lifestyle (AusDiab) Study. Am J Ophthalmol 2005;140:1157–9.

106. Diabetes Prevention Program Research Group. The prevalence of retinopathy in impaired glucose tolerance and recent-onset diabetes in the diabetes prevention program. Diabet Med 2007;24:137–44.

107. Rajala U, Laakso M, Qiao Q, et al. Prevalence of retinopathy in people with diabetes, impaired glucose tolerance, and normal glucose tolerance. Diabetes Care 1998;21:1664–9.

108. Gabir MM, Hanson RL, Dabelea D, et al. Plasma glucose and prediction of microvascular disease and mortality. Diabetes Care 2000;23:1113–8.

109. Cugati S, Cikamatana L, Wang JJ, et al. Five year incidence and progression of vascular retinopathy in persons without diabetes: the blue mountain eye study. Eye 2006;20:1239–45.

110. Van Leiden HA, Dekker JM, Moll AC, et al. Risk factors for incident retinopathy in a diabetic population, the Hoorn study. Arch Ophthalmol 2003;121:245–51.
111. Wong TY, Duncan BB, Hill Golden S, et al. Associations between the metabolic syndrome and retinal microvascular signs: the atherosclerosis risk in communities study. Invest Ophthalmol Vis Sci 2004;45:2949–54.
112. Wong TY, Mitchell P. Hypertensive retinopathy. N Engl J Med 2004;351:2310–7.
113. Ziegler D, Rathmann W, Dickhaus T, et al. Prevalence of polyneuropathy in prediabetes and diabetes is associated with abdominal obesity and macroangiopathy. Diabetes Care 2008;31:464–9.
114. Singleton JR, Smith AG. Neuropathy associated with prediabetes: what is new in 2007? Curr Diab Rep 2007;6:420–4.
115. Singelton JR, Smith AG, Bromberg MB. Increased prevalence of impaired glucose tolerance in patients with painful sensory neuropathy. Diabetes Care 2001;24:1448–53.
116. Sumner CJ, Sheth S, Griffin JW, et al. The spectrum of neuropathy in diabetes and impaired glucose tolerance. Neurology 2003;60:108–11.
117. Panzer C, Lauer M, Brieke A, et al. Association of fasting plasma glucose with heart recovery in healthy adults. Diabetes 2002;51:803–7.
118. Putz Z, Tabak AG, Toth N, et al. Noninvasive evaluation of neural impairment in subjects with impaired glucose tolerance. Diabetes Care 2009;32:181–3.
119. Vincent AM, Hinder LM, Pop-Busui R, et al. Hyperlipidemia: a new therapeutic target for diabetic neuropathy. J Peripher Nerv Syst 2009;14:257–67.
120. Barr EL, Wong TY, Tapp RJ, et al. Is peripheral neuropathy associated with retinopathy and albuminuria in individuals with impaired glucose metabolism? Diabetes Care 2006;29:1114–6.
121. Green AQ, Krishnan S, Finucane FM, et al. Altered c-fiber function as an indicator of early peripheral neuropathy in individuals with impaired glucose tolerance. Diabetes Care 2010;33:174–6.
122. Costa LA, Canani LH, Lisboa HR, et al. Aggregation of features of the metabolic syndrome is associated with increased prevalence of chronic complications in type 2 diabetes. Diabet Med 2004;21:252–5.
123. Pop-Busui R, Sima A, Stevens M. Diabetic neuropathy and oxidative stress. Diabetes Metab Res Rev 2006;22:257–73.

Pathophysiology of Prediabetes

Ele Ferrannini, MD[a],*, Amalia Gastaldelli, PhD[b], Patricia Iozzo, MD[b]

KEYWORDS

- Prediabetes • Insulin resistance • β-cell dysfunction
- Dysglycemia • Hyperinsulinemia

Whatever the definition of prediabetes may be, at present or in the future, its pathophysiology is a direct extension of the physiology of glucose control. In fact, all evidence indicates that progression to diabetes occurs along a continuum, not necessarily linear with time, of glucose concentration and mechanisms; plasma glucose thresholds, on the other hand, are practical clinical constructs, generally used for diagnosis and treatment. Therefore, it is appropriate, and equivalent, to describe the pathophysiology of prediabetes both in terms of continuous changes in glucose parameters and as shifts in glucose tolerance category.

The glucose system is highly homeostatic, swinging in plasma glucose concentrations rarely exceeding 3 mmol/L (54 mg/dL) in normal people. At any given time, the plasma glucose concentration represents a balance between entry of glucose into and exit from the circulation via cellular metabolism or excretion; excessive release or defective removal (or combinations of the two) results in increasing glucose levels. Entry and exit of glucose are subject to multiple regulatory mechanisms, with insulin and glucagon principally controlling entry and insulin governing exit. The pathophysiology of prediabetes can therefore be reduced to the following questions: Is glucose release abnormal? If so, is it because of changes in β-cell or α-cell function or hepatic sensitivity to these hormones? Is glucose disposal abnormal? If so, is it caused by β-cell dysfunction or changes in peripheral tissue sensitivity to insulin? Are there relationships between glucose release and removal?

A preliminary consideration is the unique organization of the insulin/glucagon system. For many protein and nonprotein hormones, action is modulated by at least 1, often 2, hierarchical hormonal feedback pathway (eg, corticotropin-releasing hormone and adrenocorticotropic hormone for cortisol, gonadotropin-releasing hormone and gonadotropins for sex steroids). In these cases, sensitivity is provided by the circulating hormone concentrations acting on specific hormone receptors

The authors have nothing to disclose.
[a] Department of Internal Medicine, University of Pisa School of Medicine, Via Roma, 67, 56100 Pisa, Italy
[b] CNR Institute of Clinical Physiology, Via Moruzzi, 1, 56100 Pisa, Italy
* Corresponding author.
E-mail address: ferranni@ifc.cnr.it

Med Clin N Am 95 (2011) 327–339
doi:10.1016/j.mcna.2010.11.005
0025-7125/11/$ – see front matter © 2011 Elsevier Inc. All rights reserved.

medical.theclinics.com

located on target tissues as well as on the master gland of the feedback loop (eg, the pituitary). In the case of insulin and glucagon, there is no major pituitary or hypothalamic relay; target tissues control secretion directly. Thus, the circulating concentrations of substrates (mostly glucose, but also amino acids, free fatty acids [FFAs], and ketone bodies), which result from insulin action on intermediary metabolism in different tissues, feed signals back to the β-cell and the α-cell. Sensitivity gating is provided by insulin and glucagon receptors on target tissues. An additional level of regulation is paracrine in nature, ie, insulin receptors on the β-cell and the α-cell.

GLUCOSE RELEASE

Under normal circumstances of a short (10–14 hours) overnight fast, most glucose is produced by the liver,[1] with the kidney making a marginal contribution.[2] Within the liver, glucose is both synthesized, in approximately equal parts from glycogenolysis and gluconeogenesis,[3] and taken up,[4] such that what is eventually released into the bloodstream is the net sum of these simultaneous processes. With the use of labeled glucose, the amount of glucose released in the fasting state (endogenous glucose production, EGP) can be measured with acceptable accuracy. In nondiabetic healthy men and women with normal glucose tolerance (NGT) and in individuals with either impaired fasting glucose (IFG, fasting glucose between 110–126 mg/dL [6.11–7.00 mmol/L]) and a 2-hour glucose level less than 200 mg/dL (<11.1 mmol/L on a standard oral glucose tolerance test [OGTT]) or impaired glucose tolerance (IGT, fasting glucose <126 mg/dL [<7.0 mmol/L]) and a 2-hour glucose level of 140 to 199 mg/dL (7.8–11.1 mmol/L), EGP is directly and linearly related to both fat-free mass and fasting plasma glucose (FPG) concentration (**Fig. 1**). The mean values of the individuals with IFG/IGT fall to

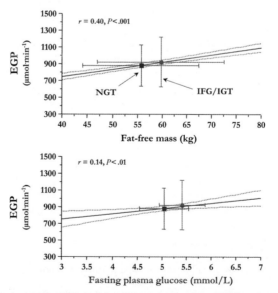

Fig. 1. Relationship between EGP and fat-free mass (*top*) and FPG concentration (*bottom*). The blue lines are best fits, and the dotted red lines are their 95% confidence intervals. Mean and standard deviation for the group with NGT (n = 355) and for the group with IFG/IGT (n = 38) are plotted. (*Unpublished data from* the RISC Study, Ferrannini E, Balkau B, Coppack SW, RISC Investigators, et al. Insulin resistance, insulin response, and obesity as indicators of metabolic risk. J Clin Endocrinol Metab 2007;92:2885–92.)

the right of those with NGT but on the same regression line. These relationships have important implications. First, EGP appears to be geared to the mass of metabolically active tissues: the larger the mass, the higher EGP. What drives this association is not known. It is possible that, as fat-free mass increases in parallel with fat mass (eg, during phases of weight gain, glucose consumption increases proportionately and minimally), chronic reductions in blood glucose levels signal the liver to rev up glucose release by autoregulation[5]; other metabolic factors, for example, circulating FFAs, may be at work (see later). Second, as individuals with IFG/IGT frequently have higher body mass index (BMI, calculated as the weight in kilograms divided by the height in meters squared) than those with NGT (28.4 vs 25.8 kg/m^2, P<.001, for the subjects in **Fig. 1**) and hence larger fat-free mass as part of their phenotype (see last section), their EGP tends to be higher, especially in individuals with IFG. As a consequence, expressing EGP in units (μmol/min) normalized for fat-free mass eliminates differences between groups (15.7 vs 16.2 μmol.min^{-1}.kg$_{ffm}$$^{-1}$, P = .67). Third, if the adaptive changes in EGP were perfect, FPG would be identical in individuals with IFG/IGT and in those with NGT. As this is not the case—fasting glycemia is significantly, if slightly, higher in individuals with IFG/IGT than in those with NGT (97 vs 90 mg/dL [5.4 vs 5.0 mmol/L], P<.0001)—the EGP response is maladaptive. The reason for this response is insulin resistance. In fact, fasting plasma insulin concentrations are significantly higher in individuals with IFG/IGT than in those with NGT (9 vs 6 μU/mL (55 vs 36 pmol/L), P<.0001), indicating that the ability of the hormone to restrain EGP is impaired. By using the product of EGP (normalized per kilogram of fat-free mass) and fasting insulin, an empiric index that has been termed insulin resistance index and used in several studies,[6] one now finds a relatively strong general relationship between glucose output and fasting glycemia (independent of body mass), along which the group with IFG/IGT are clearly separated from that with NGT (895 vs 574 μmol.min^{-1}.kg$_{ffm}$$^{-1}$ pM, P<.001) (**Fig. 2**). Once overt diabetes ensues, EGP further increases even in absolute terms, especially in poorly controlled patients.[7,8]

During absorption of a glucose load or a mixed meal, EGP is substantially suppressed in individuals with NGT,[9] significantly less so in patients with diabetes.[10] The situation in prediabetes is intermediate in that EGP is suppressed to normal absolute levels but at higher prevailing plasma insulin concentrations; calculation of a hepatic insulin resistance index under these circumstances indicates an impairment in the ability of a stimulated insulin response to adequately block postprandial glucose output.

In patients with diabetes, circulating glucagon levels are insufficiently inhibited by the hyperglycemia and hyperinsulinemia that follow glucose or meal ingestion; in fact, they may increase paradoxically.[11,12] Furthermore, recent studies have shown

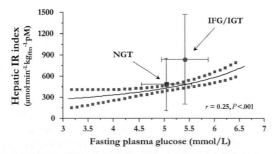

Fig. 2. Relationship between the hepatic insulin resistance (IR) index (calculated as the product of EGP and fasting plasma insulin from the data in **Fig. 1**) and FPG concentration.

that elevated fasting glucagon levels are independently associated with insulin resistance in nondiabetic individuals.[13] This finding can be interpreted as evidence that the α-cell, which is richly equipped with insulin receptors, is less responsive to the inhibitory influence of the hormone in states of generalized insulin resistance such as prediabetes.[14] The hepatic sensitivity to glucagon, on the other hand, has been reported to be preserved in patients with type 2 diabetes and presumably is similarly intact in prediabetes, although the relative contribution of glycogenolysis and gluconeogenesis to EGP may be shifted in favor of the latter as a source of circulating glucose.[15]

With regard to glucose uptake, the liver takes up circulating glucose (as does the gut), but its contribution to overall glucose disposal, as assessed by the hepatic vein catheterization technique[4] and, more recently, by positron emission tomography with ¹⁸F-fluorodeoxyglucose (¹⁸FDG-PET),[16] is limited in humans. Although sensitive to insulin,[17] the liver mainly responds to hyperglycemia by a mass action effect.[4,18] Studies using ¹⁸FDG-PET have shown that insulin-mediated glucose uptake by the liver is impaired in patients with type 2 diabetes, in proportion to the severity of hyperglycemia[19]; presumably, a lesser extent of impairment is present in prediabetes, although this has not been directly determined in these patients. In contrast to glucose, the liver extracts 2 to 3 times more circulating FFA (especially shorter-chain FFA[20]) than resting muscle (as measured by PET [positron emission tomography] and ¹⁸F-6-thia-heptadecanoic acid[21]). Although liver FFA uptake is slightly reduced in patients with IGT,[22] hepatic oxidation of this substrate is increased in obese patients.[23] Because prediabetic individuals are often overweight or obese, enhanced liver fat oxidation is likely another metabolic feature of prediabetes. FFAs do not contribute net carbon to de novo glucose synthesis, but their oxidation stimulates the activity of key gluconeogenic enzymes (pyruvate carboxylase, phosphoenolpyruvate carboxykinase, glucose-6-phosphatase) as well as provides the energy for the process.[24] Furthermore, FFA inhibit liver glycolysis,[25] thereby completing an intrahepatic substrate competition cycle analogous to the one described by Randle[26] in isolated skeletal muscle. The prediction that an augmented availability of FFA results in a reduction in liver glucose uptake has in fact been verified in PET studies using an exogenous lipid infusion to increase FFA delivery to the liver.[27]

In summary, in the liver of the prediabetic patients, insulin resistance is manifested as a reduced ability of insulin to restrain glucose release, especially from gluconeogenesis, and to stimulate glucose uptake. Enhanced FFA flux, uptake, and oxidation compete with glycolysis and stimulate gluconeogenesis, thereby adding a purely metabolic component to the cellular defects in insulin action.[28] In recent years, it has become evident that body fat distribution is an additional factor in the control of EGP (and in general, of liver function). Independent of total body fat mass, accumulation of adipose tissue within the visceral/abdominal region and the liver is associated with an accentuation of insulin resistance of gluconeogenesis.[29] Inflammatory changes in adipose depots and consequent release of inflammatory cytokines are probable mechanisms for this effect.[30]

GLUCOSE DISPOSAL

When assessed by the euglycemic clamp technique (and expressed as the total amount of glucose used normalized by fat-free mass as well as steady-state clamp insulin concentrations [M/I]), insulin sensitivity is found to be progressively impaired from NGT to IFG to IGT to overt type 2 diabetes (**Fig. 3**). To emphasize the continuous nature of the relationship between insulin sensitivity and glucose tolerance, **Fig. 4**

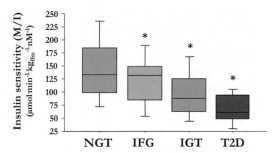

Fig. 3. Insulin sensitivity (as box plots of the M/I) in individuals with NGT, impaired fasting glucose (IFG), IGT, and type 2 diabetes (T2D). Asterisks indicate a significant difference from the NGT group. (*Data from* the RISC Study, Ferrannini E, Balkau B, Coppack SW, RISC Investigators, et al. Insulin resistance, insulin response, and obesity as indicators of metabolic risk. J Clin Endocrinol Metab 2007;92:2885–92.)

shows the regression of M/I on the OGTT 2-hour plasma glucose concentration adjusted for gender, age, and BMI; all else being equal, M/I decreases by approximately 11 units per each mmol/L increase in 2-hour plasma glucose concentrations. Thus, peripheral insulin resistance is a central metabolic feature of prediabetes independent of factors, such as gender, age, and obesity, which themselves affect insulin action. Even within the realm of NGT, individuals with higher glucose increments during a standard dynamic test such as the OGTT are more insulin resistant than those whose glucose excursions are lower. Ethnicity may contribute to insulin resistance independent of glucose tolerance and other determinants. In a study using the insulin clamp technique, Mexican-Americans were shown to be more insulin resistant than non-Hispanic whites, regardless of whether they were with NGT, IGT, or diabetes.[31]

With regard to the tissues responsible for impaired insulin-mediated glucose uptake, skeletal muscle dominates because it typically represents approximately 40% of body weight.[32] However, adipose tissue makes a significant contribution to whole body glucose disposal, as demonstrated by an [18]FDG-PET study,[33] especially in an overweight phenotype as the prediabetic individual. Moreover, in the adipocyte,

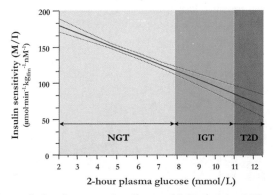

Fig. 4. Reciprocal association between insulin sensitivity (as the M/I) and 2-hour plasma glucose concentration on a standard OGTT. The relation shown by the solid line and its 95% confidence intervals is adjusted for center, sex, age, and BMI. T2D, type 2 diabetes. (*Data from* the RISC Study, Ferrannini E, Balkau B, Coppack SW, et al, RISC Investigators. Insulin resistance, insulin response, and obesity as indicators of metabolic risk. J Clin Endocrinol Metab 2007;92:2885–92.)

insulin resistance of glucose uptake limits the availability of α-glycerophosphate, which is necessary for FFA reesterification, resulting in excessive FFA net release into the bloodstream. In turn, the augmented delivery of FFA to insulin target tissues causes their preferential uptake over that of circulating glucose, thereby realizing the classical Randle cycle.[26] In fact, studies combining indirect calorimetry with the clamp technique[34] have demonstrated that lipid oxidation rates are increased and glucose oxidation rates are correspondingly decreased in insulin-resistant individuals both in the fasting state and during insulinization (clamp or OGTT), a phenomenon that has been later renamed metabolic inflexibility.[35] In the heart, this chronic shift in substrate use imposes a preferential use of FFAs, which are more oxygen costly than glucose as a fuel,[36] a demand that may be undesirable under ischemic conditions.[37] Another consequence of insulin resistance on glucose oxidation is an increase in the accumulation of lactate in the circulation, a hallmark of ischemia, and reduced glycogen accumulation.[34]

Of note is that peripheral insulin resistance is influenced by fat distribution in the same negative direction as hepatic insulin resistance.[33] It is therefore not surprising that peripheral and hepatic insulin resistances, when expressed in appropriate units, are found to be quantitatively related to one another (**Fig. 5**), as is also the case between skeletal and myocardial muscles.[36] IFG and IGT differ somewhat in the relative severity of hepatic versus peripheral insulin sensitivity, the hepatic insulin sensitivity being worse in IFG, peripheral insulin sensitivity in IGT.[38] However, this distinction is rather tenuous because IFG is associated with IGT in more than 60% of the cases; isolated IFG is rare in the population and carries little population attributable risk for diabetes.[39]

β-CELL FUNCTION

Plasma glucose concentrations increase minimally even in the presence of profound insulin resistance as long as the β-cell response is adequate; the hyperglycemia that defines prediabetes ensues when some critical aspect of β-cell function becomes defective. The normal β-cell adaptive response to insulin resistance is an upregulation of its set point: at each plasma glucose concentration absolute insulin secretion rates, both in the fasting state and throughout an OGTT, are higher in insulin-resistant individuals than in insulin-sensitive individuals. In prediabetic individuals, the relationship between insulin secretion and insulin sensitivity is a similar curvilinear function as in

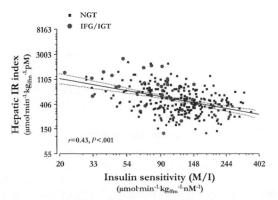

Fig. 5. Log-log plot of the relationship between the hepatic insulin resistance (IR) index and insulin sensitivity (as the M/I) for the subjects in **Fig. 1**.

those with NGT, only shifted upward as a result of their higher plasma glucose levels (**Fig. 6**). The higher plasma glucose levels, therefore, are not explained by a deficiency in the absolute amount of secreted insulin. The cause of hyperglycemia is the reduced ability of the β-cell to respond to increasing glucose levels in a timely fashion during stimulation, which is clearly shown when plotting insulin secretion rates against concomitant glucose levels: for each increment in glucose concentration during an OGTT insulin secretion is less in prediabetic states than in NGT states (**Fig. 7**). Analogous to the concept of insulin resistance, the slope of the relationship between insulin secretion and glucose concentration is an expression of β-cell glucose sensitivity.[40] Once again, the mechanism represents a continuum, from NGT to diabetes through prediabetes.[41]

This dynamic aspect of β-cell function is crucial for 2 reasons: (1) it is largely independent of insulin sensitivity and (2) it is tightly linked with glucose tolerance (**Fig. 8**).[42] In fact, in the RISC study database[43] both insulin resistance and β-cell glucose insensitivity are independently associated with IFG/IGT: in a mutiple logistic regression model adjusting for sex, age, and BMI, an M/I value in the lowest quartile of its distribution carries an odds ratio of 3.7 (with a 95% confidence interval of 2.4–5.7), while a value of β-cell glucose sensitivity in the bottom quartile carries an odds ratio of 5.1 (95% confidence interval: 3.5–7.6). Individuals falling into the bottom 25% of both physiologic variables have a 9-fold increase in the likelihood of being prediabetic. The codominant role of insulin resistance and β-cell glucose insensitivity in predicting incident dysglycemia has been confirmed in an observational follow-up study of a cohort enriched with individuals with a family history of diabetes.[44]

It should be noted that empiric indices of β-cell function, such as the acute insulin response to intravenous glucose (AIR)[45,46] and the insulinogenic index on the OGTT,[40,42] have also been used to signal defective β-cell function in prediabetes. Although qualitatively related to β-cell glucose sensitivity, these indices are much less sensitive in discriminating IFG/IGT from NGT (see **Fig. 8**).

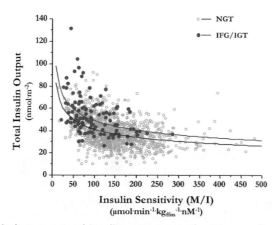

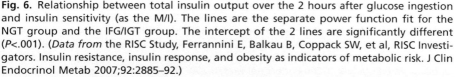

Fig. 6. Relationship between total insulin output over the 2 hours after glucose ingestion and insulin sensitivity (as the M/I). The lines are the separate power function fit for the NGT group and the IFG/IGT group. The intercept of the 2 lines are significantly different (*P*<.001). (*Data from* the RISC Study, Ferrannini E, Balkau B, Coppack SW, et al, RISC Investigators. Insulin resistance, insulin response, and obesity as indicators of metabolic risk. J Clin Endocrinol Metab 2007;92:2885–92.)

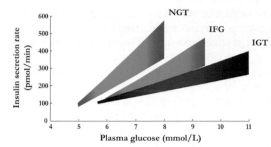

Fig. 7. Insulin secretion rates against concomitant plasma glucose concentrations during a standard OGTT. The color areas encompass mean and standard error of the slope calculated for the 3 groups by mathematical modeling. (*Data from* Ferrannini E, Mari A. Beta cell function and its relation to insulin action in humans: a critical appraisal. Diabetologia 2004;47:943–56.)

If numerically unrelated, the two main pathophysiologic defects responsible for the loss of glucose tolerance, that is, insulin resistance and β-cell glucose insensitivity, tend to occur together in prediabetes as well as overt diabetes and to covary consensually over time.[44] It has therefore been natural to ask the question, whether there is a structural link or cause-and-effect relationship between them. Knocking out insulin receptors selectively in β-cells impairs glucose sensing of the isolated perfused pancreata from these mice.[47] More recent studies have indicated that insulin potentiates

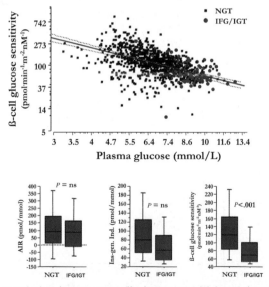

Fig. 8. Reciprocal association between β-cell glucose sensitivity and mean plasma glucose level during an OGTT (*upper panel*). For the NGT and IFG/IGT groups, the lower panel shows (as box plots) values for the acute insulin response (AIR) to intravenous glucose, the insulinogenic index (ratio of insulin-to-glucose increments 30 minutes into the OGTT), and β-cell glucose sensitivity measured in the same group. The group difference is only significant for the measure of β-cell glucose sensitivity. (*Data from* the RISC Study, Ferrannini E, Balkau B, Coppack SW, et al, RISC Investigators. Insulin resistance, insulin response, and obesity as indicators of metabolic risk. J Clin Endocrinol Metab 2007;92:2885–92.)

glucose-stimulated insulin secretion in vivo in healthy humans.[48] The precise cellular mechanisms linking insulin signaling to glucose sensing in the β-cell remain to be clarified, as do the in vivo circumstances under which this interaction becomes important.

THE CLINICAL PHENOTYPE

The abnormalities of glucose concentrations and their determinants are part of a constellation of subclinical abnormalities that consistently occur together in prediabetic individuals. As compiled in **Fig. 9**, in comparison with NGT controls, patients with IFG/IGT have a higher family history of diabetes, are slightly more often men than women, are somewhat older, are definitely heavier, and have a more central distribution of body fat; values of heart rate and systolic and diastolic blood pressures are higher as are serum lipid levels (low-density lipoprotein cholesterol, triglycerides, and FFA), whereas high-density lipoprotein cholesterol concentrations are lower, and hyperinsulinemia is present both in the fasting state and 2 hours after glucose ingestion. Importantly, the strong association between insulin resistance and β-cell glucose insensitivity with prediabetes resists statistical adjustment for the lipid and hemodynamic abnormalities as well as familial diabetes. This finding supports the notion that the genetic imprint conveyed by familial diabetes is phenotypically specified as the pathophysiologic mechanisms of hyperglycemia. In fact, multiple common

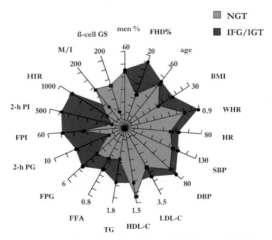

Fig. 9. Mean clinical and metabolic characteristics of NGT and IFG/IGT individuals. The data are arranged as graduated spokes, each representing a variable, along which the blue square plots the mean value of the NGT group and the black dot that of the IFG/IGT group; the profile results from connecting the 2 series of dots and filling it in light blue for the NGT group and in red for the IFG/IGT group. The variables are men %, percentage of male subjects; FHD %, percentage of persons with a positive family history of diabetes; age (in years); BMI (in kg/m²); WHR, waist-to-hip ratio; HR, heart rate; SBP, systolic blood pressure; DBP, diastolic blood pressure; LDL-C, low-density lipoprotein cholesterol in mmol/L; HDL-C, high-density lipoprotein cholesterol in mmol/L; and TG, triglycerides in mmol/L; FFAs in mmol/L; FPG; 2-h PG, 2-hour plasma glucose on the OGTT in mmol/L; FPI, fasting plasma insulin; 2-h FPI, 2-hour fasting plasma insulin on the OGTT in pmol/L; HIR, hepatic insulin resistance index; M/I, insulin sensitivity from the clamp technique; and β-cell GS, β-cell glucose sensitivity from mathematical modeling of the OGTT. (*Data from* the RISC Study, Ferrannini E, Balkau B, Coppack SW, et al, RISC Investigators. Insulin resistance, insulin response, and obesity as indicators of metabolic risk. J Clin Endocrinol Metab 2007;92:2885–92.)

variants of type 2 diabetes genes are associated with defects in β-cell function.[49,50] The clustering also suggests that insulin resistance/hyperinsulinemia may link diabetes with clinical hypertension and dyslipidemia either mechanistically or by genetic linkage (or both).

Recent work has emphasized that the phenotype in **Fig. 9** is closely predictive of nonalcoholic fatty liver disease.[51] A meta-analysis of available evidence has concluded that prediabetes per se (IFG, IGT, or both combined) is associated with a modest but significant increase in risk for cardiovascular disease.[52]

SUMMARY

Prediabetes encompasses conventional diagnostic categories of IFG and IGT (or, in the future, HbA_{1c}[53]) with thresholds subject to change, but actually is a band of glucose concentrations and a temporal phase over a continuum extending from conventional NGT to overt type 2 diabetes. Insulin resistance, at the level of the liver and peripheral tissues, and defective glucose sensing at the β-cell are the central pathophysiologic determinants that together cause and predict the defining hyperglycemia. Regardless of the cellular origin of the insulin resistance, excessive tissue fat utilization is a consistent metabolic mechanism. Although genetic influences affect β-cell function, becoming overweight is the main acquired challenge to insulin action.[54] The phenotype of prediabetes includes dyslipidemia and higher arterial blood pressure, thereby representing a common soil of atherogenic risk.

REFERENCES

1. Ferrannini E, Groop LC. Hepatic glucose production in insulin-resistant states. Diabetes Metab Rev 1989;5:711–26.
2. Meyer C, Stumvoll M, Dostou J, et al. Renal substrate exchange and gluconeogenesis in normal postabsorptive humans. Am J Physiol Endocrinol Metab 2002;282:E428–34.
3. Gastaldelli A, Baldi S, Pettiti M, et al. Influence of obesity and type 2 diabetes on gluconeogenesis and glucose output in humans: a quantitative study. Diabetes 2000;49:1367–73.
4. DeFronzo RA, Ferrannini E, Hendler R, et al. Regulation of splanchnic and peripheral glucose uptake by insulin and hyperglycemia in man. Diabetes 1983;32: 35–45.
5. Bolli G, De Feo P, Perriello G, et al. Role of hepatic autoregulation in defense against hypoglycemia in humans. J Clin Invest 1985;75:1623–31.
6. Natali A, Toschi E, Camastra S, et al. Determinants of postabsorptive endogenous glucose output in non-diabetic subjects. European Group for the Study of Insulin Resistance (EGIR). Diabetologia 2000;43:1266–72.
7. DeFronzo RA, Simonson D, Ferrannini E. Hepatic and peripheral insulin resistance: a common feature of type 2 (non-insulin-dependent) and type 1 (insulin-dependent) diabetes mellitus. Diabetologia 1982;23:313–9.
8. Woerle HJ, Szoke E, Meyer C, et al. Mechanisms for abnormal postprandial glucose metabolism in type 2 diabetes. Am J Physiol Endocrinol Metab 2006; 290:E67–77.
9. Ferrannini E, Bjorkman O, Reichard GA Jr, et al. The disposal of an oral glucose load in healthy subjects. A quantitative study. Diabetes 1985;34:580–8.
10. Ferrannini E, Simonson DC, Katz LD, et al. The disposal of an oral glucose load in patients with non-insulin-dependent diabetes. Metabolism 1988;37:79–85.

11. Reaven GM, Chen YD, Golay A, et al. Documentation of hyperglucagonemia throughout the day in nonobese and obese patients with noninsulin-dependent diabetes mellitus. J Clin Endocrinol Metab 1987;64:106–10.
12. Muscelli E, Mari A, Casolaro A, et al. Separate impact of obesity and glucose tolerance on the incretin effect in normal subjects and type 2 diabetic patients. Diabetes 2008;57:1340–8.
13. Ferrannini E, Muscelli E, Natali A, et al. Relationship between Insulin Sensitivity and Cardiovascular Disease Risk (RISC) Project Investigators. Association of fasting glucagon and proinsulin concentrations with insulin resistance. Diabetologia 2007;50:2342–7.
14. Gromada J, Franklin I, Wollheim CB. A-cells of the endocrine pancreas: 35 years of research but the enigma remains. Endocr Rev 2007;28:84–116.
15. Nielsen MF, Wise S, Dinneen SF, et al. Assessment of hepatic sensitivity to glucagon in NIDDM: use as a tool to estimate the contribution of the indirect pathway to nocturnal glycogen synthesis. Diabetes 1997;46:2007–16.
16. Iozzo P, Jarvisalo MJ, Kiss J, et al. Quantification of liver glucose metabolism by positron emission tomography: validation study in pigs. Gastroenterology 2007;132:531–42.
17. Iozzo P, Geisler F, Oikonen V, et al, 18F-FDG PET Study. Insulin stimulates liver glucose uptake in humans: an 18F-FDG PET Study. J Nucl Med 2003;44:682–9.
18. Alzaid AA, Dinneen SF, Turk DJ, et al. Assessment of insulin action and glucose effectiveness in diabetic and nondiabetic humans. J Clin Invest 1994;94:2341–8.
19. Iozzo P, Hallsten K, Oikonen V, et al. Insulin-mediated hepatic glucose uptake is impaired in type 2 diabetes: evidence for a relationship with glycemic control. J Clin Endocrinol Metab 2003;88:2055–60.
20. Hagenfeldt L, Wahren J, Pernow B, et al. Uptake of individual free fatty acids by skeletal muscle and liver in man. J Clin Invest 1972;51:2324–30.
21. Iozzo P, Turpeinen AK, Takala T, et al. Liver uptake of free fatty acids in vivo in humans as determined with 14(R, S)-[18F]fluoro-6-thia-heptadecanoic acid and PET. Eur J Nucl Med Mol Imaging 2003;30:1160–4.
22. Iozzo P, Turpeinen AK, Takala T, et al. Defective liver disposal of free fatty acids in patients with impaired glucose tolerance. J Clin Endocrinol Metab 2004;89:3496–502.
23. Iozzo P, Bucci M, Roivainen A, et al. Fatty acid metabolism in the liver, measured by positron emission tomography, is increased in obese individuals. Gastroenterology 2010;139(3):846–56, e1–6. Available at: http://www.ncbi.nlm.nih.gov/pubmed/20685204Gastroenterology. Accessed May 25, 2010.
24. Ferrannini E, Barrett EJ, Bevilacqua S, et al. Effect of fatty acids on glucose production and utilization in man. J Clin Invest 1983;72:1737–47.
25. Hue L, Maisin L, Rider MH. Palmitate inhibits liver glycolysis. Involvement of fructose 2,6-bisphosphate in the glucose/fatty acid cycle. Biochem J 1988;251:541–5.
26. Randle PJ. Regulatory interactions between lipids and carbohydrates: the glucose fatty acid cycle after 35 years. Diabetes Metab Rev 1998;14:263–8.
27. Iozzo P, Lautamaki R, Geisler F, et al. Non-esterified fatty acids impair insulin-mediated glucose uptake and disposition in the liver. Diabetologia 2004;47:1149–56.
28. Kahn CR, Folli F. Molecular determinants of insulin action. Horm Res 1993;39(Suppl 3):93–101.
29. Gastaldelli A, Miyazaki Y, Pettiti M, et al. Separate contribution of diabetes, total fat mass, and fat topography to glucose production, gluconeogenesis, and glycogenolysis. J Clin Endocrinol Metab 2004;89:3914–21.

30. Olefsky JM, Glass CK. Macrophages, inflammation, and insulin resistance. Annu Rev Physiol 2010;72:219–46.
31. Ferrannini E, Gastaldelli A, Matsuda M, et al. Influence of ethnicity and familial diabetes on glucose tolerance and insulin action: a physiological analysis. J Clin Endocrinol Metab 2003;88:3251–7.
32. Ferrannini E, Mari A. How to measure insulin sensitivity. J Hypertens 1998;16: 895–906.
33. Virtanen KA, Iozzo P, Hällsten K, et al. Increased fat mass compensates for insulin resistance in abdominal obesity and type 2 diabetes: a positron-emitting tomography study. Diabetes 2005;54:2720–6.
34. Golay A, DeFronzo RA, Ferrannini E, et al. Oxidative and non-oxidative glucose metabolism in non-obese type 2 (non-insulin-dependent) diabetic patients. Diabetologia 1988;31:585–91.
35. Kelley DE. Skeletal muscle fat oxidation: timing and flexibility are everything. J Clin Invest 2005;115:1699–702.
36. Paternostro G, Camici PG, Lammerstma AA, et al. Cardiac and skeletal muscle insulin resistance in patients with coronary heart disease. A study with positron emission tomography. J Clin Invest 1996;98:2094–9.
37. Iozzo P, Chareonthaitawee P, Dutka D, et al. Independent association of type 2 diabetes and coronary artery disease with myocardial insulin resistance. Diabetes 2002;51:3020–4.
38. Abdul-Ghani MA, Tripathy D, DeFronzo RA. Contributions of beta-cell dysfunction and insulin resistance to the pathogenesis of impaired glucose tolerance and impaired fasting glucose. Diabetes Care 2006;29:1130–9.
39. Ferrannini E, Massari M, Nannipieri M, et al. Plasma glucose levels as predictors of diabetes: the Mexico City diabetes study. Diabetologia 2009;52:818–24.
40. Ferrannini E, Mari A. Beta cell function and its relation to insulin action in humans: a critical appraisal. Diabetologia 2004;47:943–56.
41. Ferrannini E, Gastaldelli A, Miyazaki Y, et al. Beta-cell function in subjects spanning the range from normal glucose tolerance to overt diabetes: a new analysis. J Clin Endocrinol Metab 2005;90:493–500.
42. Mari A, Tura A, Natali A, et al, RISC Investigators. Impaired beta cell glucose sensitivity rather than inadequate compensation for insulin resistance is the dominant defect in glucose intolerance. Diabetologia 2010;53:749–56.
43. Ferrannini E, Balkau B, Coppack SW, et al, RISC Investigators. Insulin resistance, insulin response, and obesity as indicators of metabolic risk. J Clin Endocrinol Metab 2007;92:2885–92.
44. Walker M, Mari A, Jayapaul MK, et al. Impaired beta cell glucose sensitivity and whole-body insulin sensitivity as predictors of hyperglycaemia in non-diabetic subjects. Diabetologia 2005;48:2470–6.
45. Brunzell JD, Robertson RP, Lerner RL, et al. Relationships between fasting plasma glucose levels and insulin secretion during intravenous glucose tolerance tests. J Clin Endocrinol Metab 1976;42:222–9.
46. Kahn SE, Zraika S, Utzschneider KM, et al. The beta cell lesion in type 2 diabetes: there has to be a primary functional abnormality. Diabetologia 2009; 52:1003–12.
47. Otani K, Kulkarni RN, Baldwin AC, et al. Reduced beta-cell mass and altered glucose sensing impair insulin-secretory function in betaIRKO mice. Am J Physiol Endocrinol Metab 2004;286:E41–9.
48. Bouche C, Lopez X, Fleischman A, et al. Insulin enhances glucose-stimulated insulin secretion in healthy humans. Proc Natl Acad Sci U S A 2010;107:4770–5.

49. Pascoe L, Tura A, Patel SK, et al, RISC Consortium. U.K. Type 2 Diabetes Genetics Consortium. Common variants of the novel type 2 diabetes genes CDKAL1 and HHEX/IDE are associated with decreased pancreatic beta-cell function. Diabetes 2007;56:3101–4.

50. Pascoe L, Frayling TM, Weedon MN, et al, RISC Consortium. Beta cell glucose sensitivity is decreased by 39% in non-diabetic individuals carrying multiple diabetes-risk alleles compared with those with no risk alleles. Diabetologia 2008;51: 1989–92.

51. Gastaldelli A, Kozakova M, Højlund K, et al, RISC Investigators. Fatty liver is associated with insulin resistance, risk of coronary heart disease, and early atherosclerosis in a large European population. Hepatology 2009;49:1537–44.

52. Ford ES, Zhao G, Li C. Prediabetes and the risk for cardiovascular disease: a systematic review of the evidence. J Am Coll Cardiol 2010;55:1310–7.

53. Fonseca V, Inzucchi SE, Ferrannini E. Redefining the diagnosis of diabetes using glycated hemoglobin. Diabetes Care 2009;32:1344–5.

54. Ferrannini E. Insulin resistance versus insulin deficiency in non-insulin-dependent diabetes mellitus: problems and prospects. Endocr Rev 1998;19:477–90.

Diagnosis of Prediabetes

Jonathan Shaw, MD, FRACP, FRCP(UK)

KEYWORDS
- Prediabetes • Impaired glucose tolerance
- Impaired fasting glucose • Diagnosis • Risk score

Among people with prediabetes, the risk of developing diabetes can be markedly reduced with both lifestyle and pharmacologic interventions (see the article by Ratner and Sathasivam elsewhere in this issue for further exploration of this topic). Putting these interventions into place necessitates a careful, reasoned, and cost-effective approach to identifying those with prediabetes. A variety of diagnostic tools have been used to identify prediabetes. Most of these tools depend on blood glucose levels, but others identify high risk of diabetes through risk equations accounting for other risk factors. This article reviews these diagnostic approaches, with the aim of describing how they identify individuals at the greatest risk of developing diabetes and diabetes-related outcomes.

CAN PREDIABETES BE DIAGNOSED?

Before addressing the issue of how to diagnose prediabetes, it is necessary to consider the somewhat philosophic question of whether diagnosis is the correct or appropriate term. The term diagnosis has typically been reserved for categorization or identification of individuals with a distinct disease. Because the term disease implies a condition that causes symptoms (dis-ease), prediabetes has not usually been considered to be a disease[1] and therefore cannot be diagnosed. Although prediabetes is widely considered to be asymptomatic, it is noteworthy that at least one study has shown that quality of life is impaired in prediabetes.[2] Nevertheless, prediabetes is considered to be a risk state, rather than a disease, and therefore, the term diagnosis is somewhat inappropriate. This terminology has implications beyond philosophy and semantics because the degree of certainty required to diagnose a disease is typically greater than that required for assigning risk. Hence, the diagnosis of diseases often requires tests for confirmation of the diagnosis, but this recommendation is not made for assessing risk. Thus, the diagnosis of diabetes or hypertension requires abnormal readings on more than 1 day, but this method does not apply to the calculation of Framingham risk score. The corollary is that unless and until prediabetes is considered to be a disease in its own right, identification of those people with

Baker IDI Heart and Diabetes Institute, Level 4, 99 Commercial Road, Melbourne 3004, Australia
E-mail address: jonathan.shaw@bakeridi.edu.au

Med Clin N Am 95 (2011) 341–352
doi:10.1016/j.mcna.2010.11.012
0025-7125/11/$ – see front matter © 2011 Elsevier Inc. All rights reserved.

medical.theclinics.com

prediabetes, by whichever means (blood glucose level testing or risk factor scores), will not need additional confirmatory tests.

IMPAIRED FASTING GLUCOSE AND IMPAIRED GLUCOSE TOLERANCE

As detailed in the article by Buysschaert and Bergman elsewhere in this issue, in the last several decades, there has been a series of modifications in the blood glucose levels considered to be diagnostic of diabetes. Much debate has focused on the relative merits of impaired fasting glucose (IFG) and impaired glucose tolerance (IGT) as predictors of both diabetes and cardiovascular disease (CVD); the evidence to this debate is summarized in this article. Although IFG and IGT share many similarities, the degree to which they represent the principal pathophysiologic aspects of hyperglycemia (muscle and liver insulin resistance, insulin secretory deficits) differs (see the article by Ferrannini and colleagues elsewhere in this issue), and hence, the associations of IFG and IGT with diabetes and CVD might be expected to differ. Practical issues are also important—IFG can be determined from a single fasting blood test, whereas IGT requires a 2-hour oral glucose tolerance test (OGTT). Thus, any recommendation to include consideration of diagnosing IGT as well as (or instead of) IFG must recognize the practical challenges its measurement entails.

Glucose level, like most other risk factors for diabetes and CVD, has a continuous relationship with the risk of diabetes or CVD.[3,4] This is important to recognize when trying to compare IGT with IFG in regard to prediction of diabetes and CVD. The categories of IFG and IGT (particularly in regard to their lower cut points) represent relatively arbitrary sections on the continuum of risk between glucose levels and these outcomes. Inevitably, therefore, in studies examining the risks associated with IFG or IGT compared with a low-risk group (using relative risk or odds ratio), the findings are partially dependent on the reference category used (ie, whether the category is fasting plasma glucose [FPG]<110 mg/dL, or 2-hour plasma glucose [2hPG]<140 mg/dL, or FPG<110 mg/dL and 2hPG<140 mg/dL). Therefore, even if FPG and 2hPG values had identical risks of CVD and diabetes, the relative risk of IFG compared with FPG less than 110 mg/dL could be different to the relative risk of IGT compared with 2hPG less than 140 mg/dL, simply because the 2 reference categories did not have the same risk as each other.

When attempting to examine glucose level as an independent risk factor for CVD or total mortality, a common approach to accounting for the lack of power in individual studies is to combine data from several studies.[5] Although combining data addresses the issues of power well, it also brings an important limitation. Differences between studies in the methods of glucose measurement, such as the type of blood sample (whole blood vs plasma or capillary blood) and glucose assay method, inevitably introduce imprecision into an assessment of the relationship between glucose level or glucose category and outcomes. The imprecision may be particularly relevant when considering narrow categories such as IFG, because a small variation in blood glucose measurements can frequently make the difference between an individual being classified or not classified within the category.

Finally, although the focus is usually on the extent to which a relationship between glucose level and an outcome is independent of known or potential confounders (such as other CVD risk factors), both unadjusted and adjusted relationships between glucose level and outcomes have utility. For example, glucose level may have value as a risk marker for CVD even if this relationship is mediated through its association with other CVD risk factors. A special example is whether the relationship between FPG and outcomes is independent of 2hPG and vice versa.

IFG and IGT as Predictors of Diabetes

In a systematic review of IFG and IGT, Santaguida and colleagues[6] assessed the properties of both in relation to predicting new-onset diabetes. Across more than 40 studies of people with IFG and IGT, they reported a wide range of annual incidence of diabetes from 1.6 to 34.0 per 100 persons per year. The variations reflect the influence of other nonglycemic diabetes risk factors such as ethnicity[7] and age.[8] When considering the risk of developing diabetes compared with the normal reference group (which varies in definition from study to study, see earlier discussion), **Fig. 1** shows that the highest risk was for those individuals with combined IFG and IGT. The risks associated with IGT seemed to be higher than those associated with IFG, but the overlapping confidence intervals (CIs) suggest that this difference is not statistically significant. This higher risk associated with IGT is consistent with data from a large Australian study,[9] published after the review by Santaguida and colleagues, but in the review by Santaguida and colleagues,[6] among 3 studies that reported risks for both IFG and IGT, the risk seemed to be higher for IFG than for IGT.

From a population perspective, sensitivity and specificity for diabetes are at least as important as risk (or positive predictive value). The sensitivity of IFG as originally defined (FPG = 110–125 mg/dL) is less than that of IGT in most populations,[10] but the specificity of IFG is somewhat greater.[11] IGT identifies a larger number of individuals who will ultimately develop diabetes, largely because IGT is more common than IFG (with a lower limit of 110 mg/dL) in most populations. Not surprisingly, these differences are entirely dependent on the cut points selected and not on any inherent differences between FPG and 2hPG.[12] When categorized in groups containing equal proportions of the population, abnormalities of FPG or 2hPG had the same predictive values for subsequent diabetes.[12] When the lower limit of IFG is reduced to 100 mg/dL, the sensitivity of IFG increases to approximately that of IGT, but the specificity decreases.

Thus, neither the risk of developing diabetes nor the sensitivity and specificity for diagnosing diabetes seem to differ enough between IGT and IFG to merit the

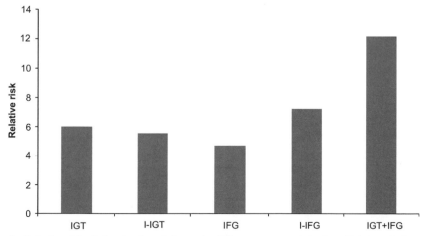

Fig. 1. Relative risk of developing diabetes in different categories of prediabetes. Reference group is those with normal glucose tolerance (defined in each study). I-IGT, isolated IGT; I-IFG, isolated IFG; IGT + IFG, combined IFG and IGT. (*Data from* Santaguida PL, Balion C, Hunt D, et al. Diagnosis, prognosis, and treatment of impaired glucose tolerance and impaired fasting glucose. Evid Rep Technol Assess (Summ) 2005;128:1–11.)

superiority of one over the other. However, because in most populations IGT is much more common than IFG (if IFG is defined as FPG = 110–125 mg/dL), it identifies a greater proportion of those who will develop diabetes. Furthermore, even if IFG is defined as FPG = 100–125 mg/dL and therefore has a prevalence that is much closer to that of IGT, the 2 groups remain limited in their overlap. Therefore, performing an OGTT to identify those with IGT identifies a greater proportion of the at-risk population than can be achieved by simply relying on FPG.

In most longitudinal studies, 20% to 40% of those individuals who develop diabetes have normal glucose tolerance at baseline. Because all individuals pass through the stage of prediabetes before developing diabetes, this percentage is largely dependent on the interval between baseline and follow-up (the longer the study, the more likely it is that new cases of diabetes at follow-up were normal at baseline) and on the rate at which an individual's blood glucose level increases. Regarding the latter, an analysis of a UK study[13] showed that individuals who ultimately developed diabetes displayed a gradual increase in both FPG and 2hPG measurements over approximately 10 years, followed by a more rapid increase over the 3 years immediately preceding diabetes onset.[14] This highlights the fact that a measurement of fasting and 2HPG at a single point in time is of limited utility in identifying all those at risk of developing diabetes within a population. Taking additional risk factors into account may improve this method and is considered later.

IFG and IGT as Predictors of CVD

In addition to the well-known association between diabetes and CVD, prediabetes is also associated with CVD. Indeed, there is a continuous relationship between blood glucose levels and CVD, which extends well into the normal range.[3,4,15] In recognizing the importance of CVD as an outcome of both diabetes and prediabetes, ascertaining which manifestation of prediabetes (IFG or IGT) better predicts the development of CVD may be helpful in guiding practice in relation to diagnosing prediabetes. Should IGT be shown to be clearly superior to IFG in predicting CVD, a strong case could be made for using IGT as the main clinical diagnostic tool, because interventions based on the presence of IGT are more likely to reduce the burden of CVD than those based on the presence of IFG.

The data relating prediabetes to CVD have been reviewed by Ford and colleagues.[16] A total of 27 longitudinal studies were included, reporting on IFG defined with a lower limit of 100 mg/dL (IFG 100) or 110 mg/dL (IFG 110) and on IGT.

Data from 175,000 participants in 18 publications were available for IFG 110. Increased risks of CVD were reported in 15 of 18 publications but were statistically significant in only 7 of these 15 publications. Considering all 18 publications, the overall relative risk of developing CVD for people with IFG 110 was 1.20 (95% CI, 1.12–1.28). Not surprisingly, the relative risk reported in those studies that adjusted for other CVD risk factors was lower than in studies not adjusted for these risk factors, but the difference was not statistically significant (1.12 vs 1.24, $P = .129$), and the risk of developing CVD was only of marginal statistical significance in those studies adjusting for other risk factors. IFG 110 possibly conveyed a greater risk among women than men (relative risks, 1.30 vs 1.17, respectively), although this difference was not statistically significant.

There were 8 publications providing information on IFG 100 in 53,000 participants, all were adjusted for other CVD risk factors. Among the 8 publications, 7 reported an increased risk of CVD for people with IFG 100, although results were statistically significant in only 2 individual publications. Overall, a statistically significant increased risk of 18% was found (relative risk 1.18; 95% CI, 1.09–1.28). Unlike IFG 110, the risk of

CVD associated with IFG 100 seemed to be slightly higher in men than in women, but again, the differences were not statistically significant.

Data from 54,000 participants on the relationship between IGT and CVD were reported in 8 publications. All but 2 of the 8 publications reported an increased risk associated with IGT, but only 1 publication reported statistically significant results. Overall, a statistically significant increased risk of 20% was found (relative risk 1.20; 95% CI, 1.07–1.34), with risks being no different in the 6 publications adjusted for other CVD risk factors than in the 2 that did not. There were 4 publications that appropriately used both the FPG and the 2hPG criteria to define IGT. These 4 publications had the lowest CVD risks, and together, they showed no association between IGT and CVD (relative risk 0.97; 95% CI, 0.79–1.21). Only those publications that defined IGT by 2hPG alone reported significantly increased CVD risks, suggesting that some of the risk associated with IGT may, in fact, be due to diabetes in the fasting state.

The 5 publications that reported on CVD risk in individuals with both IGT and IFG showed no significant increase in risk (relative risk 1.10; 95% CI, 0.99–1.23) when compared with people with normal glucose tolerance.

It has often been speculated that the CVD risks reported in relation to IFG and IGT are manifested in only those who subsequently develop diabetes; therefore, the risks are a consequence of diabetes but not a direct consequence of prediabetes. However, in the small number of studies that have attempted to examine this issue, the results are conflicting.[17–19]

Overall, it seems that IFG and IGT have a similar and a rather modest associated excess risk of CVD. Simple comparisons of risks might lead to the conclusion that the OGTT is not justified for predicting CVD. However, there is limited overlap between the IFG and IGT populations, thus only identifying those with IFG leaves a substantial proportion of the population with prediabetes undiagnosed. Therefore, performing the OGTT is likely to identify more individuals at elevated CVD risk, who are not identified by fasting tests alone.

Diagnostic Cut Points for IFG and IGT

What is the origin and validity of the diagnostic cut points for IFG (110–125 mg/dL or 100–125 mg/dL) and IGT (140–199 mg/dL)? The upper limits are straightforward because they are the diagnostic cut points for diabetes. A detailed discussion of the upper limits is beyond the scope of this review, but data from several different sources have suggested that the diabetes diagnostic cut points are threshold values for the risk of developing retinopathy and are values that separate bimodal distributions of glucose in populations with a high prevalence of diabetes. Although there are obvious potential advantages of using CVD outcomes rather than, or as well as, retinopathy to set the diabetes diagnostic cut points, this practice has proved to be impractical. First, the continuous nature of the relationship of glucose level with CVD (as opposed to the threshold nature of the relationship with retinopathy) is not suitable to the setting of cut points. Second, from a population perspective, glucose level is a weak predictor of CVD, and adds little or nothing to Framingham risk equations,[4,20,21] and so prediction of CVD should focus on other traditional CVD risk factors.

The lower limits of IFG and IGT are less straightforward. The lower limit of IGT was set several decades ago[22] and was based primarily on data from the Pima Indians showing that with a 2hPG of more than 140 mg/dL, the risk of developing diabetes was considerably higher than for lower 2hPG values.[1] Subsequent studies have, however, shown that there is no specific cut point or threshold in this association,[12] but there has been no interest in changing what is now a well-established diagnostic value.

The lower limit of IFG was originally set at 110 mg/dL.[23] The American Diabetes Association's (ADA's) 1997 Expert Committee on the diagnosis and classification of diabetes[23] based the cut point of 110 mg/dL on several studies. First, in an analysis of the Paris Prospective Study, Charles and colleagues[24] selected a group of people just below the fasting diabetes threshold when the level was 140 mg/dL to determine whether elevated nondiabetic fasting glucose levels were comparable to IGT for predicting incident diabetes. They chose a fasting glucose cut point that would include an equal number of individuals in the new fasting category as were included in IGT. This category, defined as an FPG value of 110 to 140 mg/dL, was therefore similar to IGT, in terms of prevalence, and also proved to be similar in terms of risk of progressing to diabetes. Unfortunately, when IFG was introduced as an entity in 1997, these justifications, based on similarities with IGT, were removed by the change of the fasting diabetes cut point from 140 to 126 mg/dL. This reduction of the upper limit of IFG removed those at highest risk of progression, hence reducing its prevalence and altering its predictive characteristics.

The second strand of evidence was a small study examining insulin secretion in response to intravenous glucose administration.[25] The study indicated that the acute insulin response was lost above a FPG of 115 mg/dL. However, with only 3 participants in the category of FPG value more than 115 mg/dL (115–150 mg/dL), this analysis included far too few participants in the appropriate glucose range to provide reasonable accuracy for setting cut points. Finally, another analysis of the Paris Prospective Study showed a significant risk for coronary heart disease mortality associated with elevated but nondiabetic fasting glucose values.[26] However, the actual glucose level category associated with elevated risk was 104 to 126 mg/dL and not 110 to 125 mg/dL.

Once IFG values had been defined, data from many studies were used to examine the characteristics of the new category, especially in relation to IGT, and a series of reports demonstrated important differences between the 2 categories. IFG had a lower prevalence than IGT in virtually every population examined.[10] It also had a lower sensitivity for predicting diabetes (ie, identifying fewer individuals in the population who actually progress to developing diabetes), although maintaining a similar positive predictive value (the proportion of those with IFG who progress to diabetes and those with IGT who progress to diabetes is similar). The data further showed that there was limited overlap between IGT and the new IFG category, with only approximately 25% to 50% of individuals identified as having one of these conditions also having the other.

Recognizing the limitations of having the IFG value of 110 mg/dL as a cut point, the ADA, in 2002, reviewed all the available data on IFG to determine whether this level was optimal. 4 Longitudinal studies were identified to provide data to ascertain the FPG value that optimized the prediction of diabetes. In each of these 4 studies, the ADA examined the sensitivity and specificity of a wide range of FPG values to identify the single value that maximized the sum of sensitivity and specificity and hence came closest to providing 100% sensitivity and 100% specificity for the development of diabetes. The figure was 103 mg/dL in a Dutch population, 97 mg/dL in a Pima Indian population, 94 mg/dL in a Mauritius population, and 94 mg/dL in a San Antonio population.[27] Thus, the lower limit of IFG was changed to 100 mg/dL. Further support for lowering the cut point subsequently came from a study of more than 450 intravenous glucose tolerance test results demonstrating that first-phase insulin secretion begins to decrease once the FPG level increases above 90 to 97 mg/dL.[28]

This issue was subsequently considered by a World Health Organization (WHO) Expert Committee,[1] which elected to retain the original lower limit of 110 mg/dL. Although accepting that in relation to predicting diabetes, the sum of sensitivity and specificity was maximized at a FPG of approximately 100 mg/dL, the WHO committee did not accept that this was a sufficiently strong rationale to warrant changing the cut point, particularly because it would increase 2- to 3-fold the number of individuals with IFG. Although using this method to identify the point at which sensitivity and specificity are maximized is a common way of setting thresholds, it has significant limitations. This method assumes that sensitivity and specificity are equally important and that the implications and consequences of a false-positive case are equivalent to those of a false-negative case, which is rarely true. The WHO argued that in the absence of data showing that the new threshold identified a group in whom interventions improved outcomes, there was no justification for a change that would greatly increase the prevalence of this condition.

GLYCATED HEMOGLOBIN

Measurement of glycated hemoglobin (HbA_{1c}) levels has now been recommended for diagnosis of diabetes,[29] although it remains controversial. Levels of HbA_{1c} less than the diagnostic cut point for diabetes have recently been suggested as an alternative definition of prediabetes.[29] An International Expert Committee suggested that a person with HbA_{1c} of 6.0% to 6.5% should be considered as being at high risk for diabetes,[30] and the ADA subsequently recommended that prediabetes could be defined as an HbA_{1c} of 5.7% to 6.4%.[29] Several studies have noted a limited overlap between prediabetes defined as IGT or IFG and prediabetes defined by HbA_{1c}.[29,31] However, more important than analyses of overlap, evidence shows that (1) the risk of developing diabetes increases markedly in the HbA_{1c} range recommended by the ADA,[29] (2) HbA_{1c} is similar[9] or slightly inferior to glucose[32] in predicting diabetes, and (3) the lifestyle intervention in the Diabetes Prevention Program (in which participants with IGT were selected) was effective in those with an HbA_{1c} above and below the mean HbA_{1c} concentration of 5.9%.[29] It is noteworthy that in these studies linking HbA_{1c} to the risk of diabetes, diabetes was defined using glucose levels. Had diabetes been defined using HbA_{1c} level, it is likely that HbA_{1c} would have performed better.

As more evidence accumulates on the estimation of HbA_{1c} as a means of diagnosing diabetes, it is likely that it will be seen as offering a very similar predictive capacity as is seen with the glucose-based IGT and IFG, although having the potential for greater uptake amongst patients because it can be measured in the nonfasting state. However, the decision to use HbA_{1c} as a diagnostic tool hinges on the availability of a high-quality standardized assay and on the cost, which is typically higher than that for glucose estimation.

DIABETES RISK SCORES

Prediabetes can be viewed as a means of either describing the risks attached to elevated but nondiabetic levels of blood glucose or identifying those at the highest risk of developing diabetes. The latter approach is probably the one with the greater practical and clinical value, and therefore, blood glucose levels are not the only way to define diabetes risk. Other well-established risk factors for diabetes, such as age, ethnicity, and adiposity, can be used to construct risk tools that can also identify those at high risk. Several tools or scores, most comprising risk factors not requiring invasive testing, have been developed in recent years. However, others also include variables such as blood pressure and triglyceride levels that can only be ascertained through medical screening and are therefore confined for use within specific health care settings. These scores can be used either as a noninvasive screening tool to identify high-risk individuals requiring blood glucose measurements or as a means of using all relevant data for improving risk stratification beyond that which can be achieved with a blood glucose determination alone.

The Finnish diabetes risk score (FINDRISC)[33] is probably the most widely used and tested of these tools. Developed from prospective population-based data in Finland, it uses information on age, sex, body mass index (BMI), waist circumference (WC), physical activity, diet, use of antihypertensive drugs, history of high blood glucose level, and a family history of diabetes to estimate the absolute risk of developing diabetes over 10 years. When assessed in various populations other than the one in which the tool was developed, it has a sensitivity of 66% to 82% and a specificity of 43% to 69% for diabetes.[34] It has also been shown to be a reasonable prediction tool for CVD.[35,36] Most other noninvasive scores include similar risk factors to those included in FINDRISC. Hippisley-Cox and colleagues,[13] however, used data from a large general practice database in the United Kingdom to develop a score that included a measure of socioeconomic status and traditional risk factors.

Generalizability of Risk Scores

One important consideration for using diabetes risk scores is its applicability when used in a population differing from that in which it was developed. This consideration is particularly relevant when applying scores derived from one ethnicity to another. Glumer and colleagues[37] examined the performance of the Rotterdam Predictive Model in 9 different populations. The capacity of this diabetes risk score to identify those with undiagnosed diabetes was clearly superior in 5 predominantly Europid populations (from Europe, the United States, and Australia) compared with 4 other populations (from India, Cameroon, Korea, and Tonga). On the other hand, when several risk scores (derived from European and Thai populations) were applied to a Middle Eastern population from Oman, the differences between the scores in their capacity to identify undiagnosed diabetes were small.[38] Furthermore, the performance of these scores was not different to that of a score derived from another Omani population.[38] Thus, although it seems intuitive that scores should be restricted to populations similar to those in which they were derived, only limited data support this conclusion. It seems reasonable to assume that because ethnic groups differ greatly in their diabetes risk factor profiles, ethnic-specific or country-specific scores should be used. However, even when focusing on adiposity, which varies inversely with diabetes risk between certain ethnic groups (ie, Europids have high BMI and WC but low diabetes risk; South and South-East Asians have low BMI and WC but high diabetes risk), the relationship between adiposity and diabetes does not differ between ethnic groups. Data from cross-sectional[39] and longitudinal[40] studies have shown that for a given increase in BMI or WC, the relative increase in diabetes risk is similar in Asian and in Europid populations (**Fig. 2**). What differs is the absolute risk at any given level of BMI, which is higher for the Asian populations. Thus, developing a new score may not always require a large epidemiologic study, but calibration of an established score to the diabetes risk in the new population may suffice. This approach has yielded success in predicting CVD risk.[41]

How to Use Results of a Diabetes Risk Score

Although some have recommended that noninvasive scores can be independently used to identify those at risk of developing diabetes and they would therefore benefit from participating in a diabetes prevention program without further assessment, most guidelines recommend that those found to be at high risk based on a score should undergo blood glucose testing for definitive risk stratification. However, it is not clear whether blood glucose levels alone should then be used for risk stratification or

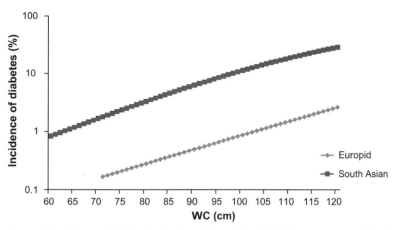

Fig. 2. Annual incidence of diabetes in Europid and South Asian men, according to WC, modeled for a 50-year-old man. (*Data from* Cameron AJ, Sicree RA, Zimmet PZ, et al. Cutpoints for waist circumference in Europids and South Asians. Obesity (Silver Spring) 2010;18(10):2039–46.)

whether these results should be used to identify those with undiagnosed diabetes, allowing the remaining high-risk individuals to participate in a diabetes prevention program. Neither of these approaches maximizes available information from blood glucose levels and the other parameters used to calculate the initial score. In recent analyses of the longitudinal population-based Australian Diabetes, Obesity and Lifestyle (AusDiab)[42] study, it was shown that after stratification with the noninvasive the Australian Diabetes Risk Score (AUSDRISK) tool and then measuring fasting blood glucose level in those at high risk, recalculating risk with a new tool that incorporated FPG as well as other noninvasive risk factors was superior to using FPG alone. These benefits were seen not only in the predictive performance of the approach but also in relation to the costs of screening and the costs of diabetes prevention.

SUMMARY

The purpose of diagnosing prediabetes is to identify a segment of the population at increased risk for the development of both diabetes and CVD so that interventions (lifestyle and pharmacologic) can be initiated. Diagnosis has traditionally been made by measuring blood glucose levels during either fasting or an OGTT. Careful analysis of longitudinal data shows that IFG and IGT are similar to each other in their ability to predict diabetes and CVD. However, because populations with IFG and IGT have limited overlap with each other, performing the OGTT to identify those with IGT provides the opportunity to identify a greater proportion of the at-risk population. HbA$_{1c}$ estimation has also been recently recommended for diagnosis of prediabetes, and although it seems to predict the development of future diabetes, its use is not yet widely accepted.

A novel approach for identifying individuals at high risk for developing diabetes is the use of simple noninvasive scores. Because these scores can predict risk without requiring medical or invasive measures, they can be easily applied to and used by the general public and offer potential for mass screening programs. Furthermore, subsequent incorporation of blood glucose results into a reconfigured score can increase the accuracy of risk prediction.

REFERENCES

1. World Health Organization. Definition and diagnosis of diabetes mellitus and intermediate hyperglycemia: report of a WHO/IDF consultation. Geneva (Switzerland): World Health Organization; 2006.
2. Tapp RJ, Dunstan DW, Phillips P, et al. Association between impaired glucose metabolism and quality of life: results from the Australian diabetes obesity and lifestyle study. Diabetes Res Clin Pract 2006;74(2):154–61.
3. Coutinho M, Gerstein H, Wang Y, et al. The relationship between glucose and incident cardiovascular events: a metaregression analysis of published data from 20 studies of 95,783 individuals followed for 12.4 years. Diabetes Care 1999;22:233–40.
4. Barr EL, Boyko EJ, Zimmet PZ, et al. Continuous relationships between non-diabetic hyperglycaemia and both cardiovascular disease and all-cause mortality: the Australian Diabetes, Obesity, and Lifestyle (AusDiab) study. Diabetologia 2009;52(3):415–24.
5. The DECODE study group. Glucose tolerance and mortality: comparison of WHO and American Diabetes Association diagnostic criteria. European Diabetes Epidemiology Group. Diabetes epidemiology: collaborative analysis of diagnostic criteria in Europe. Lancet 1999;354(9179):617–21.
6. Santaguida PL, Balion C, Hunt D, et al. Diagnosis, prognosis, and treatment of impaired glucose tolerance and impaired fasting glucose. Evid Rep Technol Assess (Summ) 2005;128:1–11.
7. Boyko EJ, Gerstein HC, Mohan V, et al. Effects of ethnicity on diabetes incidence and prevention: results of the Diabetes REduction Assessment with ramipril and rosiglitazone Medication (DREAM) trial. Diabet Med 2010;27:1226–32.
8. Knowler WC, Barrett-Connor E, Fowler SE, et al. Reduction in the incidence of type 2 diabetes with lifestyle intervention or metformin. N Engl J Med 2002; 346(6):393–403.
9. Magliano DJ, Barr EL, Zimmet PZ, et al. Glucose indices, health behaviors, and incidence of diabetes in Australia: the Australian Diabetes, Obesity and Lifestyle Study. Diabetes Care 2008;31(2):267–72.
10. Unwin N, Shaw J, Zimmet P, et al. Impaired glucose tolerance and impaired fasting glycaemia: the current status on definition and intervention. Diabet Med 2002; 19(9):708–23.
11. Shaw J, Zimmet P, Hodge A, et al. Impaired fasting glucose: how low should it go? Diabetes Care 2000;23:34–9.
12. Gabir MM, Hanson RL, Dabelea D, et al. The 1997 American Diabetes Association and 1999 World Health Organization criteria for hyperglycemia in the diagnosis and prediction of diabetes. Diabetes Care 2000;23(8):1108–12.
13. Hippisley-Cox J, Coupland C, Robson J, et al. Predicting risk of type 2 diabetes in England and Wales: prospective derivation and validation of QDScore. BMJ 2009;338:b880.
14. Tabak AG, Jokela M, Akbaraly TN, et al. Trajectories of glycaemia, insulin sensitivity, and insulin secretion before diagnosis of type 2 diabetes: an analysis from the Whitehall II study. Lancet 2009;373(9682):2215–21.
15. Brunner EJ, Shipley MJ, Witte DR, et al. Relation between blood glucose and coronary mortality over 33 years in the Whitehall Study. Diabetes Care 2006; 29(1):26–31.
16. Ford ES, Zhao G, Li C. Prediabetes and the risk for cardiovascular disease: a systematic review of the evidence. J Am Coll Cardiol 2010;55(13):1310–7.

17. Kim NH, Pavkov ME, Looker HC, et al. Plasma glucose regulation and mortality in Pima Indians. Diabetes Care 2008;31(3):488–92.
18. Qiao Q, Jousilahti P, Eriksson J, et al. Predictive properties of impaired glucose tolerance for cardiovascular risk are not explained by the development of overt diabetes during follow-up. Diabetes Care 2003;26(10):2910–4.
19. Rijkelijkhuizen JM, Nijpels G, Heine RJ, et al. High risk of cardiovascular mortality in individuals with impaired fasting glucose is explained by conversion to diabetes: the Hoorn study. Diabetes Care 2007;30(2):332–6.
20. Meigs J, Nathan D, D'Agostino R, et al. Fasting and postchallenge glycemia and cardiovascular disease risk. Diabetes Care 2002;25(10):1845–50.
21. Simmons RK, Sharp S, Boekholdt SM, et al. Evaluation of the Framingham risk score in the European Prospective Investigation of Cancer-Norfolk cohort: does adding glycated hemoglobin improve the prediction of coronary heart disease events? Arch Intern Med 2008;168(11):1209–16.
22. National Diabetes Data Group. Classification and diagnosis of diabetes mellitus and other categories of glucose intolerance. Diabetes 1979;28:1039–57.
23. American Diabetes Association. Report of the Expert Committee on the diagnosis and classification of diabetes mellitus. Diabetes Care 1997;20:1183–97.
24. Charles M, Fontbonne A, Thibult N, et al. Risk factors for NIDDM in white population. Paris Prospective Study. Diabetes 1991;40:796–9.
25. Brunzell JD, Robertson RP, Lerner RL, et al. Relationships between fasting plasma glucose levels and insulin secretion during intravenous glucose tolerance tests. J Clin Endocrinol Metab 1976;42(2):222–9.
26. Charles M, Balkau B, Vauzelle-Kervroedan F, et al. Revision of diagnostic criteria for diabetes [letter]. Lancet 1996;348:1657–8.
27. Genuth S, Alberti KG, Bennett P, et al. Follow-up report on the diagnosis of diabetes mellitus. Diabetes Care 2003;26(11):3160–7.
28. Godsland IF, Jeffs JA, Johnston DG. Loss of beta cell function as fasting glucose increases in the non-diabetic range. Diabetologia 2004;47(7):1157–66.
29. American Diabetes Association. Diagnosis and classification of diabetes mellitus. Diabetes Care 2010;33(Suppl 1):S62–9.
30. International Expert Committee. International Expert Committee report on the role of the A1C assay in the diagnosis of diabetes. Diabetes Care 2009;32(7):1327–34.
31. Mostafa SA, Khunti K, Srinivasan BT, et al. The potential impact and optimal cut-points of using glycated haemoglobin, HbA1c, to detect people with impaired glucose regulation in a UK multi-ethnic cohort. Diabetes Res Clin Pract 2010; 90(1):100–8.
32. Droumaguet C, Balkau B, Simon D, et al. Use of HbA1c in predicting progression to diabetes in French men and women: data from an Epidemiological Study on the Insulin Resistance Syndrome (DESIR). Diabetes Care 2006;29(7):1619–25.
33. Lindstrom J, Tuomilehto J. The diabetes risk score: a practical tool to predict type 2 diabetes risk. Diabetes Care 2003;26(3):725–31.
34. Schwarz PE, Li J, Lindstrom J, et al. Tools for predicting the risk of type 2 diabetes in daily practice. Horm Metab Res 2009;41(2):86–97.
35. Franciosi M, De Berardis G, Rossi MC, et al. Use of the diabetes risk score for opportunistic screening of undiagnosed diabetes and impaired glucose tolerance: the IGLOO (Impaired Glucose Tolerance and Long-Term Outcomes Observational) study. Diabetes Care 2005;28(5):1187–94.
36. Silventoinen K, Pankow J, Lindstrom J, et al. The validity of the Finnish diabetes risk score for the prediction of the incidence of coronary heart disease and stroke, and total mortality. Eur J Cardiovasc Prev Rehabil 2005;12(5):451–8.

37. Glumer C, Vistisen D, Borch-Johnsen K, et al. Risk scores for type 2 diabetes can be applied in some populations but not all. Diabetes Care 2006;29(2):410–4.
38. Al-Lawati JA, Tuomilehto J. Diabetes risk score in Oman: a tool to identify prevalent type 2 diabetes among Arabs of the Middle East. Diabetes Res Clin Pract 2007;77(3):438–44.
39. Huxley R, Barzi F, Lee CM, et al. Waist circumference thresholds provide an accurate and widely applicable method for the discrimination of diabetes. Diabetes Care 2007;30(12):3116–8.
40. Cameron AJ, Sicree RA, Zimmet PZ, et al. Cut-points for Waist Circumference in Europids and South Asians. Obesity (Silver Spring) 2010;18(10):2039–46.
41. Chen L, Tonkin AM, Moon L, et al. Recalibration and validation of the SCORE risk chart in the Australian population: the AusSCORE chart. Eur J Cardiovasc Prev Rehabil 2009;16(5):562–70.
42. Chen L, Magliano DJ, Balkau B, et al. Maximising efficiency and cost-effectiveness of type 2 diabetes screening: the AusDiab study. Diabetic Medicine 2010. [Epub ahead of print].

Diabetes Prevention Programs

A. Ramachandran, MD, PhD, DSc, FRCP (London), FRCP (Edinburgh)*,
C. Snehalatha, MSc, DPhil, DSc

KEYWORDS

- Type 2 diabetes • Primary prevention of diabetes
- Lifestyle modification • Prediabetes
- Progression to diabetes

Diabetes is a major metabolic disease that is reaching an epidemic proportion in several countries and is causing a huge health care burden. It is estimated that nearly 438 million adults worldwide will have diabetes by 2030.[1] The huge number of people with the prediabetic condition of impaired glucose tolerance (IGT) portend the future increase in prevalence of type 2 diabetes. The expected number of persons with IGT by 2030 is 472 million, a number exceeding that projected for diabetes.[1] The increasing prevalence of diabetes seen in many countries is chiefly attributed to the increase in the incidence of type 2 diabetes.[1,2] Type 2 diabetes constitutes more than 85% of all cases of diabetes worldwide, and the percentage is even higher in developing countries.[1] It is predicted that by 2030, nearly 80% of diabetic persons will be from the developing countries. Type 2 diabetes is a lifestyle disease and its escalating prevalence in developed countries is mostly attributed to aging of the population. In developing countries, increasing rates of obesity and physical inactivity and shift to unhealthy diet habits due to westernization and modernization account for the increasing incidence of the disease.

Type 2 diabetes develops because of the interaction of genetic and environmental risk factors. The recent epidemic of the disease cannot be attributed to genetic influences because these factors do not change in a short period. Therefore, marked increase in environmental risk factors caused by socioeconomic transition is the main contributory factor for the increasing prevalence of diabetes and its associated complications.

Treatment outcome in diabetes is far from optimal even in developed nations,[3] and the scenario is worse in developing nations because there are inadequate facilities and lack of awareness even among health care providers, resulting in delayed diagnosis,

The authors have nothing to disclose.
India Diabetes Research Foundation, Dr A. Ramachandran's Diabetes Hospitals, 28, Marshalls Road, Egmore, Chennai 600 008, Tamil Nadu, India
* Corresponding author.
E-mail address: ramachandran@vsnl.com

Med Clin N Am 95 (2011) 353–372
doi:10.1016/j.mcna.2010.11.006
0025-7125/11/$ – see front matter © 2011 Elsevier Inc. All rights reserved.

poor metabolic control, and widespread prevalence of complications.[4] Moreover, in several populations in developing countries, the disease develops at an early age.[5]

The Diabetes Control and Complications Trial[6]/Epidemiology of Diabetes Interventions and Complications study,[7] the UK Prospective Diabetes Study,[8] and Steno-2[9] study have demonstrated that intensive treatment of chronic hyperglycemia at the initial stage of diabetes yields beneficial outcomes that are durable for an extended period. Glycemic control instituted early in the course of diabetes seems to have a "legacy effect" (metabolic memory) that reduces the risk of vascular complications over a period.[10] Type 2 diabetes has a long latent period of dysglycemia associated with insulin resistance and a variety of cardiometabolic risk factors.[11] Moreover, the toxic effects of dysglycemia begin well before reaching the diagnostic threshold for diabetes.[12] With advancement in the understanding of the natural history, pathophysiology, and preventive strategies, it is evident that intervention should be started at the early stages of dysglycemia to achieve the desired outcome. The true cure for diabetes is probably to identify the people at risk for diabetes and prevent the functional deterioration of beta cells and insulin sensitivity by appropriate interventions.

Although there have been a few attempts in the primary prevention of type 1 diabetes, the results have not been encouraging.[13] Hence, the aspects of primary prevention of type 2 diabetes are discussed in this article.

Primary prevention is defined as the prevention of a disease by controlling modifiable risk factors through population prevention programs.[14] The nonmodifiable risk factors for type 2 diabetes are age, sex, family history of type 2 diabetes, genetic predisposition, history of gestational diabetes, and ethnicity. The modifiable risk factors include overweight and obesity, sedentary lifestyle, unhealthy diet, previously identified glucose intolerance, adverse intrauterine environment, alcohol consumption, and tobacco smoking. Modifiable risk factors are targeted by primary prevention strategies.[15]

In this article, the following aspects of primary prevention of type 2 diabetes are highlighted and discussed: (1) a description of major studies demonstrating the feasibility and effectiveness of primary prevention strategies in type 2 diabetes, (2) a comparative assessment of the studies using lifestyle modification (LSM) and pharmacologic agents, (3) mechanism of action of the intervention strategies, (4) collateral benefits of the prevention strategies on cardiovascular risk factors, and (5) economics of prevention strategies.

SELECTION OF STUDIES FOR THE REVIEW

Systematic randomized prospective studies of primary prevention of type 2 diabetes using LSM or pharmacologic agents with a minimum follow-up for 2 years are described. The authors have referred to reviews on primary prevention of type 2 diabetes published since 2006. A Cochrane review[16] and a monogram printed in the 6th World Congress on Prevention of Diabetes and its complications[17] have also been referenced. The study materials have been collected from diabetes journals and PubMed. Publications by the World Health Organization, International Diabetes Federation, and American Diabetes Association have also been referred.

FEASIBILITY AND EFFECTIVENESS OF PRIMARY PREVENTION STRATEGIES IN TYPE 2 DIABETES

Diabetes prevention programs (DPPs) conducted in different parts of the world in various ethnic and racial populations have conclusively shown that type 2 diabetes is a preventable disease. By controlling the adverse effects of environmental risk factors either by LSM[18–23] or with pharmacologic agents,[20,21,24,25] the development of diabetes in people at high risk for the disease can be prevented or delayed considerably. Persons with IGT and/or impaired fasting glucose (IFG) or women with a history of gestational diabetes have high risk for diabetes and have been studied in all the long-term trials.

Primary prevention studies are broadly classified as downstream, midstream, or upstream programs.[26] Downstream programs target individuals having the highest risk of disease (persons with IGT or IFG). Midstream programs target defined populations or communities found to be at increased risk of diabetes (eg, Pima Indians, Asian Indians). Upstream programs target the whole population and include public policy and environmental interventions intended to increase the support for maintaining a healthy lifestyle.

The high-risk approach (downstream strategy) is the most practical for primary prevention. For identification of high-risk subjects, the risk score assessment has been found to be simple and economical because the cost of screening by blood tests in large numbers can be avoided. It also helps to identify new cases of diabetes and subjects with other components of metabolic syndrome, such as dyslipidemia and hypertension. The risk scores are race and ethnic specific and need to be validated for individual populations.[27]

Hoorn Study

This population-based cohort study showed that although individuals with IGT or IFG at baseline constituted only 16% of the population, at the end of a 6-year follow-up, they contributed to more than 60% of the new cases of diabetes.[28]

Major Primary Prevention Studies Using LSM

LSM is found to be effective in subjects of varied ethnicity, in men and women, and in overweight[19,20] or lean subjects.[18,21,23] Racial variations in effectiveness are seen. Prevention of type 2 diabetes requires lifestyle changes related to physical activity, diet, and behavior. Healthy diet, regular physical exercise, and avoidance of smoking and excess alcohol consumption are emphasized. The principles of LSM are sustained physical activity of 30 to 40 minutes on all or a minimum of 5 days a week and restricted calorie intake, with reduction of refined carbohydrate and fat content and inclusion of food fiber.[17] Reduction of weight in obese persons by intensive practice of LSM has shown beneficial effects.

Table 1 shows the details of the major diabetes prevention studies that used LSM as an intervention.

Malmö Feasibility Study

The study done in Malmö, Sweden, was one of the earliest studies that showed that lifestyle intervention could reduce the incidence of diabetes in men with IGT or normal glucose tolerance (NGT).[29] The lifestyle advice included exercise training and diet modification, and the results were compared with a nonrandomized group receiving no intervention. In a 6-year period, LSM resulted in a significant reduction ($P<.001$) in the incidence of diabetes. More importantly, a 12-year follow-up analysis showed that mortality in the intervention group with IGT was lower than in those receiving standard care (6.5 and 14.0, respectively, per 1000 person-years; $P = .009$).[30]

The China Da Qing Study

The study was conducted in 577 people with IGT from 33 participating clinics, using cluster randomization.[18] The participants were randomized to 4 groups who were

Table 1
Major primary prevention studies in diabetes using LSM

Study (Year) (References)	Randomization Procedure Sample Size (n) Ethnic Group	Duration of Intervention	Mean Age (y) Mean BMI (kg/m²)	Inclusion Criteria	Control Group	Intervention Groups Strategies	Compliance Measure	Behavioral Intervention	Outcomes Primary	Outcomes Secondary	Relative Risk Reduction (%)	Hazard Ratio (95% CI)
Da Qing (1997)[18]	Cluster n = 577 Asian (Chinese)	Mean, 6 y	45 26	FPG <140 mg/dL (<7.8 mmol/L) or 2h PG <200 mg/dL (<11.1 mmol/L)	General instructions for diet and/or increased leisure PAs	PA: encouraged to increase physical exercise; duration dependant on intensity and counseling similar to diet only and exercise only intervention groups Diet: if BMI <25, 25–30 kcal/kg with 55%–65%; carbohydrate, 10%–15%	Exercise and diet: quantified using standardized forms and interviews 3d food record	Not reported	Incident diabetes	FPG, 2h PG, mortality	PA: 31 PA + diet: 46 Diet: 42	0.61 (0.38, 0.98)
DPS (2001)[19]	Stratified by center, sex, and 2h PG value n = 523 Finnish	Mean, 3.2 y	55 31.1	Age 40–64 y BMI >25 Kg/m² IGT 2h PG: 7.8–11.0 mmol/L FPG <7.8 mmol/L	General written and oral information to prevent diabetes mellitus at baseline and annually	PA + diet: individual counseling regarding moderate activity for 30 min/d; supervised strength training; frequency and availability varied among study centers. Low-fat high-fiber diet; goal BMI<25 or 5–10 kg weight loss; <50% carbohydrate, <30% fat, <300 m	Monitored by individual interviews at each linial visit 3d food records	Food records; goal setting	Incident diabetes	FPG, 2h PG, Wt, BMI, waist, WHR, lipids, BP cost	58	0.74 (0.54, 1.01)

DPP (2002)[20]	Adaptive randomization, n = 3234 White (54.7%), African American (19.9%), Hispanic (15.7%), American Indian (5.3%), Asian (4.4%)	Median, 2.8 y (range, 1.8–4.6 y)	50.6	34	BMI >24 FPG 95–125 mg/dL (5.2–6.9 mmol/L) and 2h 75 g OGTT PG 140–199 mg/dL (7.8–11.0 mmol/L)	Placebo: written information and annual 30-min individual session on LSM	PA + diet: moderate-intensity exercise for 150 min/wk; supervised group exercise sessions twice a week were offered 7% weight loss through a healthy low-calorie low-fat diet	Measuring percentage of participants achieving the goal of weight loss of 7% PA: assessed from logs kept by the participants	Culturally sensitive materials and motivational strategies	Incident diabetes, cardiovascular disease	FPG, Wt, BMI, waist, WHR, BP, cost mortality — 58 — 0.50 [0.42, 0.59]
IDPP (2006)[21]	Consecutive n = 531 Asian (Indian)	Median, 30 mo	45.9	25.8	Age 35–55 y IGT 2h PG 7.8–11.0 mmol/L (140–199 mg/dL) FPG <7.0 mmol/L (<126 mg/dL)	Standard health care advice at baseline	PA + diet: sedentary or light PA, participants encouraged PA for at least 30 min/d. Reduction in intake of total calories, refined carbohydrates, and fats; inclusion of fiber-rich foods	Adherence self-reported, based on weekly pattern	Motivational strategies	Incident diabetes	FPG, 2h PG, Wt, BMI, waist, lipids, BP, mortality — 28.5 — 0.74 (0.57, 0.96)
Kosaka Japanese trial (2005)[23]	4:1 assignment n = 484 Asian (Japanese)	4 y	51.5	23.9	FPG <140 mg/dL 2h PG 140–199 mg/dL	For BMI ≥24, 5%–10% smaller meals and increased PA For BMI <24, diet and exercise	PA + diet: to maintain BMI = 22, reduce food intake by 10%, avoid fat and alcohol, moderate exercise of 30–40 min/dy or 30 min cycling in weekends	Not reported	Encourage cooperation of family members, goal setting Repeated motivation at 2–3 mo interval	Incident diabetes	Wt — 67.4 — —

BMI (body mass index) calculated as the weight in kilograms divided by height in meters squared.

Abbreviations: BP, blood pressure; CI, confidence interval; DPS, Diabetes Prevention Study; FPG, fasting plasma glucose; OGTT, oral glucose tolerance test; PA, physical activity; PG, plasma glucose; WHR, waist to hip ratio; Wt, weight.

prescribed (1) a regulated diet, (2) increased physical activity, (3) diet regulation and improved physical activity, or (4) no intervention (control). At the 6-year follow-up period, all 3 interventions were equally effective in reducing the conversion to diabetes when compared with the control group (see **Table 1**).

A 20-year follow-up analysis performed in 2006 showed that the combined intervention group had a 43% lower incidence of diabetes, controlled for age and clustering by clinic, than the control group, thus demonstrating the long-lasting benefits of LSM for the prevention of diabetes (**Table 2**).[31]

The Finnish Diabetes Prevention Study

This study randomized 522 overweight persons with IGT into 2 groups: the control group, which received advice on general healthy lifestyle at the baseline visit, and the intervention group, which received individualized advice and behavioral support.[19] The goals of the intervention were body weight reduction of 5% or more; total fat intake of less than 30% of energy, with saturated fat intake of less than 5%; fiber intake of 15 g/1000 cal; and moderate exercise of at least 30 minutes per day. At the end of a 3-year follow-up, a 58% relative risk reduction in diabetes was noted (see **Table 1**). It was noteworthy that among those who achieved all the lifestyle goals, none developed type 2 diabetes.

The DPP

This trial was conducted in a multiethnic population of the United States and randomized 3234 adults with IGT, originally in 4 groups: placebo control group, LSM group, metformin group, and troglitazone group. The troglitazone group was withdrawn within a year because of the adverse effect of the drug.[20] A healthy, low-calorie, low-fat diet and physical activity of moderate intensity were advised. LSM training was given by case managers to the participants assigned to the LSM group, with 74% achieving the goal of 150 minutes or more of activity per week at 24 weeks. The results showed that intensive diet and exercise intervention reduced incident diabetes by 58%, patients followed up for a mean duration of 2.8 years, when compared with the control group. Effectiveness of metformin was less than that of LSM (relative risk reduction of 31%). Most of the effect was explained by the change in body weight.[32]

The Indian DPP

Prevention of diabetes is of utmost importance in India, the country that is likely to have the highest number of diabetic persons in the world for the foreseeable future.[1,2,21,22] The escalating prevalence of diabetes in India and other South Asian countries could be related to the rapid urbanization and socioeconomic transition causing adverse environmental effects on an existing genetic predisposition.[5] The Indian DPP (IDPP) 1[21] was designed with the aim of determining whether primary prevention of diabetes was feasible in the Asian Indian population who were younger, leaner, and more insulin resistant than the White population.

IDPP-1 was a community-based randomized controlled study in 531 participants with persistent IGT (421 men and 110 women). Their mean age (45.9 ± 5.7 years) and body mass index (BMI, calculated as the weight in kilograms divided by height in meters squared; 25.8 ± 3.5 kg/m^2) were similar to those of the Chinese cohort in the Da Qing study[18] but were significantly lower than those in the DPP[20] and Diabetes Prevention Study (DPS)[19] cohorts. The 4 arms of the study were (1) control with standard advice, (2) LSM of moderate intensity, (3) treatment with metformin (250 mg twice a day), and (4) a combination of LSM and metformin therapy. The details of randomization and outcome are shown in **Table 1**.

In a median follow-up period of 30 months, the rate of conversion to diabetes was high in the control group (18.3% per year). The relative risk reductions were similar in all 3 individual interventions (approximately 29%). Combination intervention with LSM and metformin was equally effective in reducing the incidence of diabetes, and there were no additional benefits by combining both.

Importantly, the beneficial changes in glycemia and basic pathophysiology occurred without significant weight reduction.

IDPP-2[22] was another community-based, placebo-controlled, 3-year, prospective study in which 407 participants with persistent IGT were randomized to either LSM and 30 mg of pioglitazone or LSM and placebo. The aim was to find out whether combination with pioglitazone would enhance the effectiveness of LSM. At the end of 3 years, the cumulative incidence of diabetes in the placebo (31.6%) and the pioglitazone (29.8%) arms was similar (adjusted hazard ratio of 1.084 [95% confidence interval, 0.753–1.560]; $P = .665$). Normoglycemia was achieved in 32.3% and 40.9% participants who received placebo and pioglitazone, respectively ($P = .109$).

There was no additional benefit on glycemic outcome by combining pioglitazone with LSM. The most probable explanation for this observation was that the maximum possible benefit on pathophysiology was produced by LSM and no additional improvement could occur by adding an insulin sensitizer.

The result of IDPP-2 was at variance with that of the Diabetes REduction Assessment with ramipril and rosiglitazone Medication (DREAM) study,[24] which showed a significant relative risk reduction in incident diabetes with pioglitazone therapy in participants with IGT and/or IFG. An ethnicity-related difference in the action of pioglitazone in nondiabetic persons may have been responsible for the divergent observation.

The Japanese Diabetes Prevention Study

A 4-year prospective study randomized 458 Japanese men with IGT to a cohort group with standard advice and an intervention group with intensive LSM that showed a relative risk reduction of 67.4% with intervention (see **Table 1**).[23] The intervention group received repeated motivation to maintain lifestyle changes and reduce BMI to less than 22 kg/m^2. Although there was a linear correlation between the incidence of diabetes and the BMI, the reduction in body weight did not fully account for the beneficial effect.

STUDIES USING PHARMACOLOGIC AGENTS
Early Studies

In the Whitehall study, 204 men with IGT were randomly assigned to receive either phenformin or placebo.[33] At the end of 5 years, 181 participants were available for follow-up. The cumulative incidence of diabetes was 14% in drug-treated patients and 16% in placebo-treated patients (incident rate ratio, 0.9).[34]

The Bedford study[35] was a 10-year follow-up study comparing the outcomes of 125 participants with IGT randomized to placebo and 123 participants to tolbutamide. The cumulative incidence of diabetes after 8.5 years of follow-up was 9% in the tolbutamide group and 8% in the placebo group (incidence rate ratio, 1.1). A subsequent 10-year follow-up of these patients also failed to show any significant effect of tolbutamide on the incidence of diabetes.

Table 2
Major studies using antidiabetic agents in prevention of type 2 diabetes

Study (Year) (References)	Population	Design	Selection Criteria	Study Arms (n)		Mean Age (y)	Follow-Up (y)	Drug (Dose)	Diabetes Cumulative Incidence (%), RRR (%)	Side Effects
				Drug	Placebo/Control					
DPP (2002)[20]	White, African American, Hispanic, American Indian, Asian	Parallel, randomized, placebo controlled, open label	IGT, ADA	1073	1082	51	2.8 (mean)	Metformin (850 mg twice daily)	Placebo 11.0 Metformin 7.8 RRR 31.0	Gastrointestinal symptoms
IDPP-1 (2006)[21]	Asian	Randomized, controlled, standard care, open label	IGT, WHO	128	133	46.2	3.0 (mean)	Metformin (250 mg twice daily)	Control 55.0 Metformin 40.5 RRR 26.4	Gastrointestinal symptoms
STOP-NIDDM (2002)[25]	Multicenter	Randomized, placebo controlled, double blind	IGT, WHO	714	715	54.5	3.3 (mean)	Acarbose (100 mg thrice daily)	Placebo 42.0 Acarbose 32.0 RRR 35.8	Gastrointestinal symptoms
TRIPOD (2002)[38]	Hispanic American Women	Parallel	GDM	133	133	35	2.5 (median)	Troglitazone (400 mg/d)	Placebo 12.1 Troglitazone 5.4 (annual incidence) RRR 21.2	Hepatotoxicity

DREAM (2006)[24]	Multicenter	2 × 2 factorial, randomized, placebo controlled, double blind	IFG/IGT free of cardiovascular diseases	2635	2634	54.7	3.0 (median)	Rosiglitazone (8 mg/d)	Placebo 26.0 Rosiglitazone 11.6 RRR 60.0	Weight gain, edema
IDPP-2 (2009)[22]	Asian	Parallel, community based, randomized, placebo controlled, double blind	IGT, WHO	204	203	45.3	3.0 (mean)	LSM + pioglitazone (30 mg/d)	Placebo 31.6 Pioglitazone 29.8 RRR: no significant change	Weight gain
CANOE (2010)[42]	Canadian	Randomized, placebo controlled, double blind	IGT, ADA	103	104	NA	3.9 (median)	Combination of rosiglitazone (2 mg) and metformin (500 mg) twice daily	Placebo 39.0 Treatment 14.0 RRR 66.0	Gastrointestinal symptoms

Abbreviations: ADA, American Diabetes Association; CANOE, CAnadian Normoglycemia Outcomes Evaluation; DREAM, Diabetes REduction Assessment with ramipril and rosiglitazone Medication; GDM, gestational diabetes; IDPP, Indian DPP; RRR, relative risk reduction; STOP-NIDDM, Study to Prevent Non-Insulin-Dependent Diabetes; TRIPOD, TRoglitazone In Prevention Of Diabetes; WHO, World Health Organization.

The conclusion of these studies did not support the assertion that drug therapy could be beneficial in preventing type 2 diabetes in subjects at high risk for diabetes.

Metformin

The biguanide metformin has been extensively studied for its potential for diabetes prevention. The major studies that had included the drug were the DPP[20] study in the United States and the IDPP-1 in India.[21]

In the DPP trial,[20] 1073 participants with IGT were allocated to 850 mg of metformin twice daily therapy and 1082 to placebo. Adherence to metformin was good, and at the mean follow-up period of 2.8 years, metformin reduced the incidence of diabetes by 31% compared with placebo (see **Table 2**). Metformin was most effective in individuals who had a baseline BMI of 35 kg/m^2 or more, in whom the incidence was reduced by approximately 50%. Metformin had beneficial effects mostly in participants younger than 60 years. The mean weight loss was 1.7 kg in metformin group compared with a weight gain of 0.3 kg in the placebo group (see **Table 2**).

IDPP-1[21] showed a 26% relative risk reduction in 120 patients who used metformin at a lower dose of 250 mg twice a day. The beneficial changes were similar to those observed with LSM. IDPP-1 also demonstrated that a combination of LSM and metformin did not have an additional benefit (see **Table 2**).

A Chinese study randomized 70 participants with IGT to receive placebo or metformin at a dosage of 250 mg 3 times a day for a period of 12 months and reported a beneficial effect with the drug.[36] The incidence of diabetes was 16.2% in the placebo group compared with 3% in the metformin group.

A meta-analysis was performed on randomized trials of at least 8 weeks of metformin use compared with placebo or no treatment in nondiabetic persons.[37] Analysis of 31 trials with 4570 participants followed up for 8267 person-years showed that incidence of diabetes was reduced by 40% with an absolute risk reduction of 6%. During a mean trial duration of 1.8 years, significant improvement in body weight, lipid profile, and insulin resistance and benefit on incidence of diabetes were noted.

Acarbose—Study to Prevent Non-Insulin-Dependent Diabetes

Acarbose, an α-glucosidase inhibitor, was tested for its potential to prevent diabetes in persons with IGT in the Study to Prevent Non-Insulin-Dependent Diabetes (STOP-NIDDM) (see **Table 2**).[25] Participants (n = 1429) were randomized to either 100 mg of acarbose or a placebo, 3 times a day, for a mean period of 3.3 years. A relative risk reduction of 35.8% was seen with acarbose when compared with placebo. However, nearly one-third of those in the acarbose group could not complete the study because of gastrointestinal side effects. Therefore, the validity of the findings in a clinical setting is debated. The study also showed a 49% relative risk reduction in cardiovascular events.[25]

Thiazolidinediones

The thiazolidinediones have been used in several clinical trials for their potential to prevent type 2 diabetes. Troglitazone was the first thiazolidinedione to be tested in the primary prevention trials. The drug was found to be effective in a cohort of women with a history of gestational diabetes in the TRoglitazone In Prevention Of Diabetes (TRIPOD) study.[38] In a median follow-up period of 30 months, the drug produced a 55% risk reduction and its effect was found to persist months after drug withdrawal.

An open-labeled 3-year follow-up study with pioglitazone, instead of troglitazone, (Pioglitazone In Prevention Of Diabetes [PIPOD]) also showed results similar to those with troglitazone.[39]

In the DPP trial, troglitazone (400 mg once a day) was prescribed to 585 participants with IGT for 9 months[40] before being withdrawn due to hepatotoxicity. A remarkable reduction (75%) in the incidence of diabetes occurred in this relatively brief period.

Rosiglitazone—The DREAM trial

The DREAM trial,[24] one of the largest multicentric international drug studies conducted, tested the effectiveness of rosiglitazone and ramipril separately for the prevention of type 2 diabetes.[24] The study recruited patients with either IGT, IFG, or both (n = 5269). Rosiglitazone was highly effective in reducing the incidence of diabetes by 62%, and 50% of rosiglitazone-treated patients reverted to normoglycemia compared with 30% in the placebo group.

Rosiglitazone, like metformin in the DPP trial, seemed to be most effective in persons with a high BMI. The risk reduction in persons with BMI less than 28 kg/m^2 was 40% and 68% for BMI more than 33 kg/m^2. Several side effects such as weight gain, edema, and potential cardiovascular toxic effects[41] pose limitations for regular use of the drug in diabetes prevention.

The CAnadian Normoglycemia Outcomes Evaluation Trial

The CAnadian Normoglycemia Outcomes Evaluation (CANOE) trial randomly assigned 207 patients with IGT to receive a combination of 2 mg rosiglitazone and 500 mg metformin twice daily or matching placebo for a median period of 3.9 years. Results showed that the combination was highly effective in preventing type 2 diabetes (see **Table 2**).[42]

IDPP-2

This study tested whether a combination of pioglitazone with LSM could improve the overall efficacy of reducing the incidence of diabetes in patients with IGT.[22] As mentioned earlier, there was no additional benefit of combining the drug with LSM.

Studies Using Other Drugs

It was suggested that angiotensin-converting enzyme inhibitors might reduce the incidence of diabetes based on post hoc analysis of the Heart Outcomes Prevention Evaluation (HOPE) study[43] and also by post hoc analysis of large placebo-controlled trials.[44] The trials, including those that suggested that angiotensin II receptor blockers also may have similar effects,[45] were not designed to test diabetes prevention as the primary hypothesis, and the methodological inadequacies reduce the validity of the conclusions.[46]

A systematic review of 24 studies involving antihypertensive drugs found that diabetes incidence is unchanged or increased by thiazide diuretics and β-blockers and unchanged or decreased by angiotensin-converting enzyme inhibitors, calcium channel blockers, and angiotensin receptor blockers.[47] Overall, diabetes incidence was not a prespecified primary end point in any study, and there was insufficient evidence to definitively recommend any given antihypertensive drug class to patients at risk of developing type 2 diabetes.

In the DREAM trial, ramipril was found to be ineffective in preventing diabetes (hazard ratio, 0.9%). There was no additive effect of therapy in patients randomly assigned to ramipril plus rosiglitazone.[24]

Nateglinide; meglitinide, a rapidly acting sulfonylurea like drug; and valsartan, an angiotensin receptor blocker, were tested for their potential to prevent the development of diabetes and cardiovascular disease (CVD) among 9306 participants with IGT in the NAteglinide and Valsartan Improved Glucose Tolerance Outcomes

Research (NAVIGATOR) study.[48,49] In a median follow-up period of 4 years, neither drug nor the combination reduced the incidence of diabetes or the coprimary composite cardiovascular outcomes.

Bariatric Surgery

Pories and colleagues[50] demonstrated in a retrospective analysis that bariatric surgery can effectively reverse diabetes in obese patients. In a prospective study of patients with IGT and severe obesity, bariatric surgery was effective in significantly reducing the incidence of diabetes in comparison with an untreated control group (diabetes incidence, 0.15 cases vs 4.7 cases per 100 person-years).[51] Therefore, this methodology could be resorted to in severely obese patients.

Antiobesity Agents

Orlistat (Xenical), an antiobesity drug, was compared with placebo in the XENical in the prevention of Diabetes in Obese Subjects (XENDOS) study[52] for its potential to reduce the incidence of diabetes. With the drug versus placebo, although there was a reduction in the incidence from 9% to 6% and an associated a mean weight reduction of 2.8 kg, the results were not conclusive because of the high attrition rate (57%).

Studies in Children and Adolescents

The detrimental effects of obesity/overweight in early years of life on metabolic diseases in adults are highlighted by numerous studies.[53] A few initiatives attempting to prevent childhood obesity have shown encouraging outcomes.

A local foundation–funded extensive regional implementation of community programs for obesity prevention in El Paso, Texas, using school-based health promotion strategies, including nutrition and physical activity programs and campaigns through mass media, resulted in significant reduction in obesity among children.[54]

An 8-year DPP on body size, physical activity, and diet among children aged 6 to 11 years, in the Mohawk community, Canada, showed some success in the early part of the study in risk factor reduction. However, the benefits were not maintained over the entire 8-year period.[55] Another school-based study in the United States also found that prevention strategies did not result in greater decreases in overweight and obesity in the intervention group than the control group.[56] There was a nonsignificant reduction in the combined prevalence of overweight and obesity in both the groups (4.5% in the intervention group and 4.0% in the control group). However, the intervention did result in significantly greater reductions in various indexes of adiposity, which may reduce the risk of childhood onset of type 2 diabetes.

Benefits on Cardiovascular Risk Factors

None of the prevention studies discussed earlier were designed to study the benefits on cardiovascular events. However, some of the studies showed beneficial changes in cardiovascular risk factors. DPP reported benefits on levels of blood pressure, blood lipids, and C-reactive protein.[57,58] DPS showed benefits on levels of blood pressure, blood lipids, and plasminogen activator inhibitor 1.[19,59] With preventive measures, IDPP-1 showed beneficial changes in lipid profiles.[60]

SUSTAINABLE EFFECTS OF PREVENTION STRATEGIES

Extended phases of the China Da Qing study,[31] DPS,[61] and DPP[62] have shown that the benefits of LSM are sustained over extended periods.

The China Da Qing DPS

The first phase of the study was designed to investigate whether lifestyle interventions delivered to groups, randomized by cluster rather than by individuals, could reduce the incidence of diabetes. In the extended phase of this study, after 6 years of active study, the long-term effects in the pooled groups who received different interventions were studied for 14 years.[31] Among the 400 participants alive in 2006, 372 had investigations at hospitals or at home and 28 had only personal interviews. Review of medical records was also done. Comparisons of diabetes incidence, CVD incidence, CVD mortality, and all-cause mortality between the control and the combined intervention groups were made. Hazard rate ratios adjusted for age and clustering by clinic were determined.

The analysis showed that the intervention group had 43% lower incidence of diabetes than the control group for up to 14 years after the active intervention ceased. Onset of diabetes was delayed by an average of 3.6 years. Reduction in the overall mortality and CVD mortality rates was not statistically significant between the 2 groups.

Extended Follow-up of the Finnish DPS

The extended follow-up of the Finnish DPS assessed the extent to which the originally achieved lifestyle changes and risk reduction remained after discontinuation of active counseling.[61] After a median period of 4 years of active intervention, participants remaining free of diabetes were further followed up for a median period of 3 years, with a median total follow-up period of 7 years. During the total follow-up, the incidence of type 2 diabetes was reduced (43% risk reduction, $P = .0001$); the incidence was 4.3 and 7.4 per 100 person-years in the intervention and control groups, respectively. The risk reduction was related to the success in achieving weight loss, reduction in intake of fat, increase in dietary fiber intake, and increased physical activity. Postintervention follow-up showed a 36% relative risk reduction, indicating that the beneficial effects of lifestyle changes were maintained after discontinuation of the intervention (**Table 3**).

The DPP Outcomes Study

The original DPP trial had a mean duration of 2.8 years followed by a 10-year follow-up.[62] All active participants of the original trial were eligible for the continued follow-up. After unblinding the treatment assignments, placebo use was stopped. All participants including the original LSM group and those who had developed diabetes were offered a group-administered lifestyle curriculum. Participants in the metformin group received 850 mg of the same, twice daily, in an unblinded fashion. A total of 88% (n = 2766) enrolled for an additional median follow-up period of 5.7 years. During the extended follow-up, the LSM group partially regained weight and moderate weight loss was maintained with metformin.

Diabetes incidence in 10 years since DPP randomization was reduced by 37% in the LSM group and 18% in the metformin group when compared with placebo. The study confirmed that prevention or delay of diabetes with LSM or metformin can be maintained for at least 10 years (see **Table 3**).

The 12-Year Follow-up of the Malmö Preventive Trial

In the 12-year follow-up of 6956 men who underwent health screening at 48 years of age, mortality in the IGT intervention group was compared with an IGT nonrandomized routine treatment group, a diabetic group, and a large proportion of those with NGT.[30]

Table 3
Studies showing sustainable effect of prevention strategies

Study (References)	Follow-Up Years	Intervention (Sample Number)	Diabetes Incidence (95% CI)	Risk Reduction
DPPOS[62]	Extended, median 5.7 IQR (5.5–5.8) total 10.0 IQR (9.0–10.5)	Lifestyle (n = 910) from original LSM and n = 932 from original placebo Metformin (n = 924) 850 mg twice a day	Original LSM 5.9/100 person-years (5.1–6.8) Metformin 4.9/100 person-years (4.2–5.7) Placebo 5.6/100 person-years (4.8–6.5)	In 10 y, for lifestyle 34% (24%–42%) and for metformin 18% (7%–28%) vs placebo
Finnish DPS[61]	Extended, median 3.0 Total 7.0	N = 475, all were advised lifestyle changes	Total: intervention 4.3/100 person-years (3.4–5.4), control 7.4/100 person-years (6.1–8.9); $P = .0001$ Postintervention: intervention 4.6/100 person-years, control 7.2 $P = .0401$	In 7 y, 43% vs control 36% vs control
Da Qing Study (CDQDPS)[31]	Extended up to 14 y after active intervention	N = 568 (by interview medical records) long-term effects of active intervention assessed	Active phase Annual incidence: 7% intervention, 11% control 20 y cumulative incidence: 80% intervention, 93% control	Active phase (6 y) 51% vs control (20 y) 43% vs control

Abbreviations: CDQDPS, China Da Qing DPS; DPPOS, DPP Outcomes Study; IQR, interquartile range.

The mortality rate in the IGT intervention group was similar to that in the NGT group and was significantly lower than that in the IGT routine treatment group ($P = .009$).

It was suggested that long-term intervention with lifestyle changes reduces mortality in subjects with IGT, who had an increased risk for developing type 2 diabetes and premature mortality.

LIFESTYLE VERSUS PHARMACOLOGIC INTERVENTIONS FOR PREVENTION OF DIABETES

Lifestyle intervention was found to be an effective measure for prevention of diabetes in persons with high risk of diabetes. It was more effective than metformin in the DPP participants.[20] IDPP-1[21] found that LSM and metformin were equally effective in reducing the incidence of diabetes. There was ethnic variation in the extent of risk reduction for diabetes by treatment with LSM or drugs.[20,21]

The extended phases of the Da Qing study,[31] DPS,[61] and DPP[62] have shown that the benefits of LSM were present for a long period. On the other hand, the beneficial effects of pharmacologic agents were seen only as long as the drugs were taken. In the prevention trials in persons with IGT, the effect of metformin,[63] acarbose,[25] and troglitazone[38,40] began to dissipate shortly after withdrawal of these drugs. Therefore, it is doubtful whether treatment with antidiabetic drugs, which lower plasma glucose levels in nondiabetic individuals, can really be indicated for the prevention of type 2 diabetes.[46]

Treatment with LSM is safe and no adverse events were reported in any of the clinical trials. Moreover, it promotes behavioral changes with multiple health benefits. Treatment with LSM offers additional benefits beyond reducing plasma glucose levels.

Several adverse side effects have been reported with the use of drugs for preventing diabetes. Gastrointestinal disturbances were a major side effect of metformin[20,21] and acarbose.[25] Troglitazone produced hepatotoxic effects that led to its withdrawal from the market. Rosiglitazone in the DREAM trial[24] resulted in weight gain and edema. The drug's safety has been questioned based on its associated risk with increasing cardiovascular events.[41] The risk to benefit ratio of these agents seems to be high, and compliance to drug therapy may also be low.

Cost of treatment with LSM is less than with drugs. However, in patients who are unable to adhere to lifestyle changes, metformin is the drug of choice for prevention of diabetes.[15]

MECHANISM OF ACTION OF PREVENTIVE INTERVENTIONS

The beneficial effect of LSM in reducing the incidence of diabetes in high-risk patients has been primarily related to weight reduction in the DPP[20] trial and DPS.[19] Improvements in insulin sensitivity and beta-cell function have been reported in these studies.[19,64] In Asian populations, these benefits were independent of changes in body weight.[21,23,31] In IDPP-1, subjects with normal beta-cell function at baseline and with improved insulin sensitivity during follow-up reverted to normoglycemia, whereas deterioration in both functions led to diabetes.[65] Intervention by LSM or metformin facilitated improvement in insulin sensitivity, and thereby, demand on beta-cell function was reduced.[19,40,43,64,65] Both the PIPOD[39] and TRIPOD[38] studies showed that the drugs enhanced insulin sensitivity and preserved beta-cell function, resulting in lower rate of diabetes in comparison with placebo. In the DPP study, treatment with metformin resulted in moderate weight loss and favorable changes in insulin sensitivity, which contributed to the beneficial results in reducing the incidence of diabetes.[64]

ECONOMICS OF PREVENTION OF DIABETES

The primary goal of the prevention studies is to develop a strategy that is cost-effective and has cost-benefit when implemented in large-scale community programs. Population-based strategies are urgently needed to fight the escalating global prevalence of diabetes.

Only a few studies have addressed the cost-effectiveness of diabetes prevention. DPP[66] and IDPP-1[67] showed that LSM was more cost-effective than metformin. The DPP study group estimated that from the health care perspective, to prevent one case of diabetes in the United States, the intensive lifestyle intervention cost was $15,700 and the metformin treatment cost was $31,000.[65] Cost of prevention in DPP was high, although the overall expense to society was cost-effective.

Preventing diabetes is of enormous value for the Indian scenario because the cost of diabetes care is high. On average, an individual with diabetes spends Indian rupee (INR) Rs 10,000 (US $227) for medical care in an urban area per year.[68] In IDPP-1, the LSM cost was $1052 to prevent or delay a case of diabetes.[67] If diabetes can be prevented or delayed with LSM, the prevention program would result in a net gain in health care investment. Thus, diabetes prevention represents good use of health care resources in India and perhaps in other developing countries as well.

In the Finnish DPS, after the initial phase of 4 years of intensive lifestyle intervention, the extended phase showed an additional benefit in terms of lower risk of diabetes for at least another 3 years, without any effort from health care personnel.[61] Long-term cost-effectiveness can be improved by such an approach.

Drugs that have been effective in the prevention studies, except metformin, do not show acceptable safety profiles for long-term use. Also, they are costly and their use requires constant monitoring by health care professionals.

SUMMARY

Knowledge regarding the pathophysiology and preventive aspects of type 2 diabetes has improved substantially in the past 2 decades. Major primary prevention studies discussed in this article have conclusively demonstrated that type 2 diabetes can be prevented or at least delayed for long periods by strategies involving lifestyle change or by use of some pharmacologic agents. Lifestyle change seems to be far more advantageous, safe, and cost-effective than drugs for the prevention of diabetes. The translation of this knowledge to action at the community level is urgently needed, considering the rapid increase in the prevalence of this disease. This achievement is by no means a simple task in any country, particularly in low- and middle-income countries where disease prevalence is reaching epidemic proportions. Prevention programs need to be integrated into existing health care services and require not only involvement of the community, government, media, health care services, and education services but also financial support from national and international organizations.

REFERENCES

1. Unwin N, Whiting D, Gan D, et al, editors. IDF diabetes atlas. 4th edition. Brussels (Belgium): International Diabetes Federation; 2009. p. 22–9. Chapter 2.1.1.
2. Wild S, Roglic G, Green A, et al. Global prevalence of diabetes. Estimates for the year 2000 and projections for 2030. Diabetes Care 2004;27:1047–52.
3. Narayan KM, Zhang P, Kanya AM, et al. Diabetes: the pandemic and potential solutions. In: Jamison DT, Breman JG, Measham AR, et al, editors. Disease control priorities in developing countries. 2nd edition. New York: Oxford University Press; 2006. p. 591–603.
4. Chan JC, Gagliardino JJ, Baik SH, et al. IDMPS Investigators. Multifaceted determinants for achieving glycemic control: the International Diabetes Management Practice Study (IDMPS). Diabetes Care 2009;32:227–33.
5. Ramachandran A, Snehalatha C. Diabetes in Asia. Seminar. Lancet 2010;375: 408–18.
6. The Diabetes Control and Complications Trial research group. The effect of intensive treatment of diabetes on the development of long-term complications in insulin dependent diabetes mellitus. N Engl J Med 1993;329:977–86.
7. Nathan DM, Cleary PA, Backlund JY, et al. Diabetes Control and Complications Trial/Epidemiology of Diabetes Interventions and Complications (DCCT/EDIC)

Study Research Group. Intensive diabetes treatment and cardiovascular disease in patients with type 1 diabetes. N Engl J Med 2005;353:2643–53.

8. UK Prospective Diabetes Study (UKPDS) Group. Intensive blood glucose control with sulphonylureas or insulin compared with conventional treatment and risk of complications with subjects with type 2 diabetes (UKPDS 33). Lancet 1998; 352:837–53.

9. Gaede P, Lund-Andersen H, Parving HH, et al. Effect of a multi factorial intervention on mortality in type 2 diabetes. N Engl J Med 2008;358:580–91.

10. Holman RR, Paul SK, Bethel MA, et al. 10-year follow-up of intensive glucose control in type 2 diabetes. N Engl J Med 2008;359:1577–89.

11. Abdul-Ghani MA, William K, DeFronzo R, et al. Risk of progression to type 2 diabetes based on relationship between postload plasma glucose and fasting plasma glucose. Diabetes Care 2006;29:1613–7.

12. Gerstein HC, Pais P, Pogue J, et al. Relationship of glucose and insulin levels to the risk of myocardial infarction: a case control study. J Am Coll Cardiol 1999;33:612–9.

13. Gillespie KM. Type 1 diabetes: pathogenesis and prevention [review]. CMAJ 2006;175:165–70.

14. Rose G. Sick individuals and sick populations. Int J Epidemiol 1985;14:32–8.

15. Alberti G, Zimmet P, Shaw J. Metabolic syndrome-a new worldwide definition: a consensus statement from the International Diabetes Federation. Diabetes Metab 2006;23:469–80.

16. Orozco LJ, Buchleitner AM, Gimenez-Perz G, et al. Exercise or exercise and diet for preventing type 2 diabetes mellitus [review]. The Cochrane Collaboration and published in The Cochrane Library. Cochrane Database Syst Rev 2008;3:CD003054.

17. Lindstrom J, Tuomilehto J. The short history of diabetes prevention through lifestyle intervention. In: Schwarz PEH, Reddy P, Greaves CJ, et al, editors. Dresden WCPD. Diabetes Prevention in Practice; 2010. p. 9–18.

18. Pan X, Li G, Hu Y, et al. Effects of diet and exercise in preventing NIDDM in people with impaired glucose tolerance: the Da Qing IGT and diabetes study. Diabetes Care 1997;20:537–44.

19. Tuomilehto J, Lindstrom J, Eriksson JG, et al. Prevention of type 2 diabetes mellitus by changes in lifestyle among subjects with impaired glucose tolerance. N Engl J Med 2001;344:1343–50.

20. Knowler WC, Barrett-Conner E, Fowler SE, et al. Reduction in the incidence of type 2 diabetes with lifestyle intervention or metformin. N Engl J Med 2002;346: 393–403.

21. Ramachandran A, Snehalatha C, Mary S, et al. The Indian Diabetes Prevention Programme shows that lifestyle modification and metformin prevent type 2 diabetes in Asian Indian subjects with impaired glucose tolerance (IDPP-1). Diabetologia 2006;49:289–97.

22. Ramachandran A, Snehalatha C, Mary S, et al. Pioglitazone does not enhance effectiveness of life style modification in preventing conversion of impaired glucose tolerance to diabetes in Asian Indians-Results of Indian Diabetes Prevention Programme-2 (IDPP-2). Diabetologia 2009;52:1019–26.

23. Kosaka K, Noda M, Kuzuya T. Prevention of type 2 diabetes by lifestyle intervention: a Japanese trial in IGT males. Diabetes Res Clin Pract 2005;67:152–62.

24. Gerstein HC, Yusuf S, Holman RR, et al. Effect of rosiglitazone on the frequency of diabetes in patients with impaired glucose tolerance or impaired fasting glucose: a randomized controlled trial. Lancet 2006;368:1096–105.

25. Chiasson J, Homis R, Hanefeld M, et al. Acarbose for prevention of type 2 diabetes mellitus: the STOP-NIDDM randomized trial. Lancet 2002;359:2072–7.

26. McKinlay J. "A case for refocusing upstream: the political economy of sickness". In: Enelow A, Henderson JB, editors. Behavioural aspects of prevention. Washington, DC: American Heart Association; 1975. p. 9–25.
27. Glümer C, Vistisen D, Borch-Johnsen K, et al. Risk score for type 2 diabetes can be applied in some population but not all. Diabetes Care 2006;29:410–4.
28. Vegt FD, Dekker JM, Jager A, et al. Relation of impaired fasting and postload glucose with incident type 2 diabetes in a Dutch population. The Hoorn Study. JAMA 2001;285:2109–13.
29. Eriksson KF, Lindgard F. Prevention of type 2 non-insulin-dependent diabetes mellitus by diet and physical exercise. The 6-year Malmö feasibility study. Diabetologia 1991;34:891–8.
30. Eriksson KF, Lindgärde. No excess 12-year mortality in men with impaired glucose tolerance who participated in the Malmö Preventive Trial with diet and exercise. Diabetologia 1998;41:1010–6.
31. Li G, Zhang P, Wang J, et al. The long-term effect of lifestyle interventions to prevent diabetes in the China Da Qing Diabetes Prevention Study: a 20-year follow-up study. Lancet 2008;371:1783–9.
32. Hamman RF, Wing RR, Edelstein SL, et al. Effect of weight loss with life style intervention on risk of diabetes. Diabetes Care 2006;29:2102–7.
33. Jarrett RJ, Keen H, Fuller JH, et al. Worsening to diabetes in men with impaired glucose tolerance ("borderline diabetes"). Diabetologia 1979;16:25–30.
34. Knowler WC, Sartor G, Melander A, et al. Glucose tolerance and mortality, including a substudy of tolbutamide treatment. Diabetologia 1997;40:680–6.
35. Keen H, Jarrett RJ, Mc Cartney P. The ten-year follow-up of the Bedford survey (1962–1972): glucose tolerance and diabetes. Diabetologia 1982;22:73–8.
36. Li CL, Pan CY, Lu JM, et al. Effect of metformin on patients with impaired glucose tolerance. Diabet Med 1999;16:477–81.
37. Sally S. Meta-analysis: metformin treatment in persons at risk for diabetes mellitus. Am J Med 2008;121:149–57.
38. Buchanan TA, Xiang AH, Peters RK, et al. Preservation of pancreatic beta cell function and prevention of type 2 diabetes by pharmacological treatment of insulin resistance in high-risk Hispanic women. Diabetes 2002;51:2769–803.
39. Xiang AH, Peters RK, Kjos SL, et al. Effect of pioglitazone on pancreatic beta-cell function and diabetes risk in Hispanic women with prior gestational diabetes. Diabetes 2006;55:517–22.
40. Knowler WC, Hamman RF, Edetstein SL, et al. Diabetes Prevention Program Research Group. Prevention of type 2 diabetes with troglitazone in the Diabetes Prevention Program. Diabetes 2005;54:1150–6.
41. Nissen SE, Wolski K. Effect of rosiglitazone on the risk of myocardial infarction and death from cardiovascular causes. N Engl J Med 2007;356:2457–71.
42. Zinman B, Harris SB, Neuman J, et al. Low-dose combination therapy with rosiglitazone and metformin to prevent type 2 diabetes mellitus (CANOE trial): a double-blind randomized controlled study. Lancet 2010;376:103–11.
43. Yusuf S, Sleight P, Pogue J, et al. The Heart Outcomes Prevention Evaluation Study Investigators: effects of an angiotensin-converting–enzyme inhibitor, ramipril, on cardiovascular events in high-risk patients. N Engl J Med 2000;342:145–53.
44. Fonseca VA. Insulin resistance, diabetes, hypertension, and renin-angiotensin system inhibition: reducing risk for cardiovascular disease. J Clin Hypertens 2006;8:713–20.

45. Abuissa H, Jones PG, Marso SP, et al. Angiotensin-converting enzyme inhibitors or angiotensin receptor blockers for prevention of type 2 diabetes: a meta-analysis of randomized clinical trials. J Am Coll Cardiol 2005;46:821–6.
46. Tumilehto J. Counterpoint: evidence-based prevention of type 2 diabetes: the power of lifestyle management. Diabetes Care 2007;30:435–7.
47. Padwal R, Laupacis A. Antihypertensive therapy and incidence of type 2 diabetes: a systematic review. Diabetes Care 2004;27:247–55.
48. NAVIGATOR study group, Holman RR, Haffner SM, McMurray JJ, et al. Effect of nateglinide on the incidence of diabetes and cardiovascular events. N Engl J Med 2010;362:1463–76.
49. NAVIGATOR Study Group, McMurray JJ, Holman RR, Haffner SM, et al. Effect of valsartan on the incidence of diabetes and cardiovascular events. N Engl J Med 2010;362(16):1477–90.
50. Pories WJ, MacDonald KG Jr, Morgan EJ, et al. Surgical treatment of obesity and its effect on diabetes: 10 y follow-up. Am J Clin Nutr 1992;55(Suppl 2):582S–5S.
51. Long SD, O'Brien K, MacDonald KG Jr, et al. Weight loss in severely obese subjects prevents the progression of impaired glucose tolerance to type II diabetes: a longitudinal interventional study. Diabetes Care 1994;17:372–5.
52. Torgerson JS, Hauptman J, Boldrin MN, et al. Xenical in the prevention of diabetes in obese subjects (XENDOS) study: a randomized study of orlistat as an adjunct to lifestyle changes for the prevention of type 2 diabetes in obese patients. Diabetes Care 2004;27:155–61.
53. Ebbeling CB, Pawlak DB, Ludwig DS. Childhood obesity: public-health crisis, common sense cure. Lancet 2002;360:473–82.
54. Hoelscher DM, Kelder SH, Perez A, et al. Changes in the regional prevalence of child obesity in 4th, 8th and 11th grade students in Texas from 2000–2002 to 2004–2005. Obesity (Silver Spring) 2010;18(7):1360–8.
55. Paradise G, Levesque L, Macaulay AC, et al. Impact of diabetes prevention program on body size, physical activity, and diet among Kanien'keha:ka (Mohawk) children 6 to 11 years old: 8-year results from the Kahnawake Schools Diabetes Prevention Project. Pediatrics 2005;115:333–9.
56. Foster GD, Cooper DM, Harrell JS, et al. HEALTHY Study Group. A school-based intervention for diabetes risk reduction. N Engl J Med 2010;363(5):443–53.
57. Ratner R, Goldberg R, Haffner S, et al. Impact of intensive lifestyle and metformin therapy on cardiovascular disease risk factors in the Diabetes Prevention Program. Diabetes Care 2005;28:888–94.
58. Haffner S, Temprosa M, Crandall J, et al. Intensive lifestyle intervention or metformin on inflammation and coagulation in participants with impaired glucose tolerance. Diabetes 2005;54:1566–72.
59. Hamalainen H, Ronnemaa T, Virtanen A, et al. Improved fibrinolysis by an intensive lifestyle intervention in subjects with impaired glucose tolerance. The Finnish Diabetes Prevention Study. Diabetologia 2005;48:2248–53.
60. Snehalatha C, Mary S, Vasant V, et al. Beneficial effects of strategies of primary prevention of diabetes on cardiovascular risk factors – results of the Indian Diabetes Prevention Programme (IDPP). Diab Compl Vas Res 2008;5:25–9.
61. Lindstrom J, Ilanne-Parikka P, Peltonen M, et al. Sustained reduction in the incidence of type 2 diabetes by lifestyle intervention: the follow-up results of the Finnish Diabetes Prevention Study. Lancet 2006;368:1673–9.
62. Knowler WC, Fowler SE, Hamman RF, et al. 10-year follow-up of diabetes incidence and weight loss in the Diabetes Prevention Program Outcomes Study. Lancet 2009;374:1677–86.

63. The Diabetes Prevention Program Research Group. Effects of withdrawal from metformin on the development of diabetes in the diabetes prevention program. Diabetes Care 2003;26:977–80.
64. The Diabetes Prevention Program Research Group. Role of insulin secretion and sensitivity in the evolution of type 2 diabetes in the Diabetes Prevention Program. Effects of lifestyle intervention and metformin. Diabetes 2005;54:2404–14.
65. Snehalatha C, Mary S, Selvam S, et al. Changes in Insulin secretion and insulin sensitivity in relation to the glycaemic outcomes in subjects with impaired glucose tolerance in the Indian Diabetes Prevention Programme-1 (IDPP-1). Diabetes Care 2009;32:1796–801.
66. The Diabetes Prevention Program Research Group. Within-trial cost-effectiveness of lifestyle intervention or metformin for the primary prevention of type 2 diabetes. Diabetes Care 2003;26:2518–23.
67. Ramachandran A, Snehalatha C, Yamuna A, et al. Cost-effectiveness of the interventions in the primary prevention of diabetes among Asian Indians: within-trial results of the Indian Diabetes Prevention Programme (IDPP). Diabetes Care 2007;30:2548–52.
68. Shobana R, Rama Rao P, Lavanya A, et al. Expenditure on health care incurred by diabetic subjects in a developing country - a study from Southern India. Diabetes Res Clin Pract 2000;48:37–42.

The Economics of Diabetes Prevention

William H. Herman, MD, MPH

KEYWORDS

- Diabetes mellitus • Glucose intolerance • Cost of illness
- Health utility • Cost-effectiveness • Cost utility

In the United States, the costs associated with diabetes mellitus are increasing. The cost of medical care for people with diagnosed diabetes increased from $1 billion per year in the 1970s to $116 billion per year in 2007.[1,2] Although people with diabetes comprise less than 6% of the US population, approximately 1 in 5 health care dollars is spent caring for people with diabetes.[2] In 2007, the annual per capita health care expenditure was $11,700 for a person with diabetes and $2900 for a person without diabetes.[2] The unadjusted per capita cost ratio for a person with diabetes compared with one without diabetes is 4.0.[2] People with diabetes are older than people without diabetes, and health care costs increase with age, but even after adjusting for age, the per capita cost ratio is 2.3.[2]

Healthy lifestyle interventions for the general population and intensive lifestyle and medication interventions for high-risk individuals present opportunities for diabetes prevention. The entire population is at risk for diabetes. About 1 in 3 Americans born today will develop diabetes over the lifetime.[3] To prevent diabetes, everyone in the population should be encouraged to eat a healthy diet, be physically active, and maintain an optimal weight. This approach, termed primordial prevention, seeks to address the underlying causative risk factors for disease by changing environmental conditions and social values to encourage positive health behaviors among children, adolescents, and young adults. Observational studies have suggested that favorable and unfavorable changes in lifestyles are related to population level changes in disease burden.[4] However, a recent large clinical trial of a school-based intervention program that involved changes in the schools' food service environment and gym programs and behavioral interventions to support healthy diet and physical activity at home had only a modest effect on risk factors for type 2 diabetes.[5]

This work was supported by the Biostatistics and Economic Modeling Core of the Michigan Diabetes Research and Training Center funded by DK020572 from the National Institute of Diabetes and Digestive and Kidney Diseases.
The author has nothing to disclose.
Division of Metabolism, Endocrinology and Diabetes, University of Michigan, Brehm Tower, 6th Floor, Room 6108, 1000 Wall Street/SPC 5714, Ann Arbor, MI 48105, USA
E-mail address: wherman@umich.edu

More intensive, targeted interventions are appropriate for individuals who are at a higher risk for diabetes, including people who are old or obese or have impaired fasting glucose (IFG), impaired glucose tolerance (IGT), or HbA1c levels that indicate increased risk for future diabetes. This approach, termed primary prevention, includes screening to identify high-risk individuals and intensive lifestyle interventions that may entail substantial costs and/or the use of medications that incur costs or may in fact cause harm. Randomized, controlled clinical trials from Asia, Europe, and North America have demonstrated that treating people who have glucose intolerance with intensive lifestyle interventions or medications can delay or prevent the development of type 2 diabetes.[6–11] This article describes the costs associated with glucose intolerance and diabetes, the effect of glucose intolerance and diabetes on the quality of life, and the cost-effectiveness of screening and primary prevention interventions for diabetes prevention.

THE COSTS OF GLUCOSE INTOLERANCE AND DIABETES

The costs of medical care increase along the continuum from normal glucose tolerance to glucose intolerance to diabetes mellitus to diabetes with complications. Compared with age-matched and sex-matched people without a future diagnosis of diabetes, people destined to develop diabetes experience increased medical costs for several years before the clinical diagnosis of diabetes mellitus.[12] Costs accelerate in the 3 years before diagnosis, and in the final year before diagnosis, costs are nearly twice those of the previous year.[12] For several years before diagnosis, annual pharmacy costs are significantly greater for people who will develop diabetes, primarily related to the use of antihypertensive agents, antihyperlipidemic medications, and other cardiovascular drugs.[12] Outpatient costs for those destined to develop diabetes also increased gradually in the years before diagnosis and increased substantially in the year before diagnosis.[12] Although more variable, inpatient costs are also higher and account for most (53%) of the total additional costs.[12]

Studies that have examined costs of care in patients with IFG, IGT, or both compared with those with normal glucose tolerance have confirmed this finding. Mean annual direct medical costs are higher for persons with isolated IFG, isolated IGT, and both IFG and IGT than for normoglycemic patients.[13] In general, differences are driven by inpatient costs. Microvascular complications add almost $1900 and macrovascular complications add almost $3900 to the annual age-adjusted and sex-adjusted per-person medical costs of people with glucose intolerance compared with normoglycemic controls.[14]

The costs of medical care for people with diabetes are still higher than for people with normal glucose tolerance or glucose intolerance. In 2008, the American Diabetes Association (ADA) published a cost-of-illness study to quantify the economic burden of diabetes.[2] The direct medical cost of diabetes (costs related to the treatment of diabetes and its complications and comorbidities and general medical care) in the United States in 2007 was estimated to be $116 billion. The largest proportion of direct medical costs was incurred by people 65 years and older (56% of total direct medical costs). About 35% of the total direct medical costs were incurred by people 45 to 64 years of age and 9% by people younger than 45 years. The largest components of direct medical costs were for hospital inpatient care and nursing home care (56% of total direct medical costs). Lesser proportions were for pharmacy and supplies (24% of direct medical costs) and outpatient care (20% of direct medical costs). The ADA's descriptive cost analysis suggests that much of the direct medical cost of diabetes is incurred by older patients with long-standing diabetes and is attributable to long-term complications and comorbidities requiring hospital or nursing home care.

Additional studies have confirmed that a substantial proportion of the costs of diabetes arise from treating long-term complications, particularly cardiovascular and renal disease.[15] Per-person costs increase over baseline by more than 50% after the initiation of cardiovascular drug therapy (antihypertensives, antihyperlipidemics, digoxin, and antianginal medications) or comanagement by a cardiologist. Costs increase by 360% after a major cardiovascular event, such as stroke, myocardial infarction, revascularization procedure, or hospitalization for congestive heart failure. Abnormal renal function also increases the costs of diabetes care.[15] Microalbuminuria is associated with a 65% increase in costs, renal insufficiency (defined by estimated glomerular filtration rate <50 mL/min on at least 2 separate occasions) with a 195% increase, and end-stage renal disease (defined as long-term hemodialysis or renal transplantation) with a 771% increase.

The author's group has modeled cross-sectional data from a large population with type 2 diabetes to estimate the annual direct medical costs of care for people with glucose intolerance, diabetes, and diabetes with complications and comorbidities.[16] **Fig. 1** illustrates the annual direct medical costs for a man as he might progress from IGT to diabetes to diabetes with complications and comorbidities. With progression from IGT to diabetes treated with diet and exercise alone to diabetes treated with an oral agent to diabetes with complications and comorbidities, costs increase exponentially.

The costs of diabetic complications generally increase as a function of the duration of diabetes.[17] In an analysis that used a simulation model to project the lifetime costs of complications resulting from type 2 diabetes in the United States, macrovascular disease was the earliest and the largest cost component of the complications of diabetes, accounting for 85% of the cumulative cost of complications during the first 5 years and 52% of the costs over 30 years of diabetes. Microvascular and neuropathic complications contributed only about 15% to the cost of complications in the first 5 years of diabetes. However, there were more important contributors to the late costs of type 2 diabetes. At 30 years duration of diabetes, nephropathy accounted for 21%

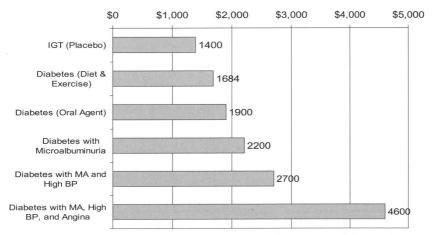

Fig. 1. Annual direct medical costs in a man progressing from IGT to diabetes with complications. (*Data from* Brandle M, Zhou H, Smith BR, et al. The direct medical cost of type 2 diabetes mellitus. Diabetes Care 2003;26:2300–4.)

of the costs of complications, neuropathy 17%, and retinopathy 10%. These results suggest that interventions to delay or prevent the development of diabetes have the potential to reduce the economic burden of cardiovascular comorbidities and delay or even prevent the costs of microvascular and neuropathic complications.

THE EFFECT OF GLUCOSE INTOLERANCE AND DIABETES ON QUALITY OF LIFE

In health economic analyses, the quality of life is assessed with the health utility score, whereby 1.0 represents perfect health and 0 represents health states equivalent to death. Scores are assigned to reflect the public's preference for each health state. In general, the quality of life decreases along the continuum from normal glucose tolerance to glucose intolerance to diabetes to diabetes with complications. A large portion of the decrement in the quality of life associated with glucose intolerance compared with normal glucose tolerance seems to be related to obesity. A study of health utility scores in an obese cohort (mean body mass index [BMI] [calculated as the weight in kilograms divided by height in meters squared], 41.8 ± 6.7) compared with an age-matched and sex-matched nonobese cohort demonstrated lower mean utility scores in the obese group for each age category.[18] In another study of patients 45 years or older, health utility scores were lower in obese patients (BMI≥30) than in normal-weight patients (BMI, 18.5–<25) even after controlling for patient characteristics (age, sex, and smoking status) and comorbidities (asthma, diabetes, stroke, heart disease, pain, arthritis, and cancer).[19]

In a study of health utility scores in people without and with type 2 diabetes, BMI was lower for patients without diabetes (27.2 ± 5.1) than for those with type 2 diabetes (28.9 ± 5.7).[20] In both the nondiabetic and type 2 diabetic patients, health utility scores were correlated with BMI and decreased with increasing BMI category (normal, overweight, obese, and extremely obese).[20] The rate of change of utility scores attributable to BMI was not significantly different between groups, even after adjusting for other known confounding factors.[20] This result suggests that both obesity and diabetes have a significant negative effect on health utility scores.

Studies have also documented decrements in health utility scores for individuals with diabetes-related complications and comorbidities. In the United Kingdom Prospective Diabetes Study (UKPDS), diabetic subjects with microvascular complications had slightly, but not significantly, lower health utility scores than diabetic patients without complications, and diabetic patients with macrovascular complications had significantly lower health utility scores than those without complications.[21] Among Dutch type 2 diabetic patients, older age, female sex, obesity, insulin therapy, and the presence of complications were associated with lower health utility scores.[22] Among Swedish patients with diabetic foot complications, those with foot ulcers and major amputations had lower health utility scores than those with primary healed ulcers.[23]

A recent study of health-related quality of life in patients with type 2 diabetes found that major diabetes-related comorbidities, including stroke and/or transient ischemic attack, hospital admission for unstable angina, myocardial infarction, and peripheral revascularization and/or amputation, had a major effect on the utility scores.[24] Minor diabetes-related comorbidities and complications, such as currently treated hypertension and diabetic eye disease, had a lesser effect.[24]

The author's group has modeled cross-sectional data from a large population with type 2 diabetes to estimate health utility scores for people with glucose intolerance, diabetes, and diabetes with complications and comorbidities.[25] **Fig. 2** illustrates the health utility scores for a man as he might progress from IGT to diabetes to diabetes

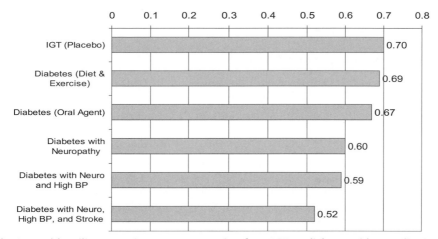

Fig. 2. Health utility scores in a man progressing from IGT to diabetes with complications. (*Data from* Coffey JT, Brandle M, Zhou H, et al. Valuing health-related quality of life in diabetes. Diabetes Care 2002;25:2238–43.)

with complications and comorbidities. With progression from IGT to diabetes treated with diet and exercise to diabetes treated with an oral agent to diabetes with complications and comorbidities, there is a progressive stepwise decrement in health utility scores.

COST-EFFECTIVENESS ANALYSIS

Cost-effectiveness analysis is a tool that compares the costs and outcomes obtained with alternative treatments and shows the difference in cost per unit of health outcome obtained.[26] It shows the economic trade-offs of one treatment strategy compared with another and provides a measure of the value obtained with alternative treatment strategies for the money spent.[26] There are 3 types of economic analyses that explicitly compare costs and outcomes.[26] They differ in how outcomes are expressed. In cost-benefit analysis, outcomes are expressed in financial terms (dollars). A limitation of cost-benefit analysis is that it is often difficult to ascribe financial value to clinical outcomes such as disease, disability, and death. In cost-effectiveness analysis, outcomes are expressed in usual clinical terms, such as cases of disease, complications, or comorbidities prevented, or years of life gained. A limitation of this method is that analyses that report different clinical outcomes cannot be directly compared. A third type of analysis that addresses the limitations of both cost-benefit and cost-effectiveness analyses is cost-utility analysis. In cost-utility analysis, the outcome is expressed with a standardized metric, the quality-adjusted life-year (QALY), which can be compared across disease states. The QALY assesses both the quality of life and length of life. QALYs are calculated as the sum of the products of the utility score for each health state times the years of life that an individual lives in each health state.

In general, cost-utility analyses are most appropriate for comparing interventions in health and medicine.[26] The cost utility of an intervention compared with that of usual care is defined as the difference in cost divided by the difference in health outcomes associated with the 2 approaches to treatment. The difference in cost is calculated as the cost associated with the intervention minus the cost associated with usual care, and the difference in health outcomes is calculated as the QALYs accrued with the intervention minus the QALYs accrued with usual care. This measure, termed the incremental cost-effectiveness ratio, provides a measure of the value obtained for the money spent.

THE COST UTILITY OF DIABETES PREVENTION

The cost utility of diabetes prevention is influenced by the cost and quality of life associated with the alternative interventions, the effectiveness of the interventions in delaying or preventing the development of diabetes and its microvascular and neuropathic complications, the effect of the interventions on cardiovascular risk factors and cardiovascular disease, the long-term safety of the interventions, and the cost and quality of life associated with the achieved health outcomes.

In the Diabetes Prevention Program (DPP), a variety of strategies were used to identify and recruit high-risk patients. The lifestyle intervention involved a healthy, low-caloric, low-fat diet and moderate physical activity, such as brisk walking. The lifestyle intervention was implemented with a 16-lesson core curriculum covering diet, exercise, and behavior modification that was taught by case managers on a one-on-one basis, followed by individual sessions (usually monthly) and group sessions with case managers. The metformin and placebo interventions were initiated at a dosage of 850 mg/d. At 1 month, the dosage of metformin or placebo was increased to 850 mg twice daily. Case managers reinforced adherence during individual quarterly sessions. All participants received standard lifestyle recommendations through written information and an annual 20- to 30-minute individual session that emphasized the importance of a healthy lifestyle.

The potential value of interventions to prevent diabetes can be best understood by reviewing the DPP Research Group's simulation of the effect of intensive lifestyle intervention and metformin on the lifetime incidence of diabetes among high-risk persons with IGT (**Fig. 3**).[27] If the entire DPP cohort were treated with the placebo intervention,

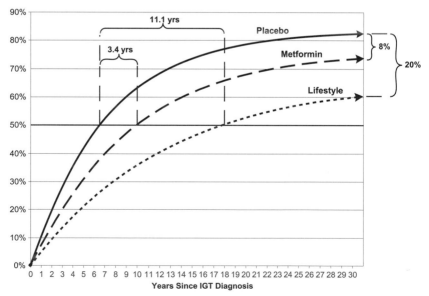

Fig. 3. Simulated cumulative incidence of diabetes in the DPP. (*From* Herman WH, Hoerger TJ, Brandle M, et al. The cost-effectiveness of lifestyle modification or metformin in preventing type 2 diabetes in adults with impaired glucose tolerance. Ann Intern Med 2005;142:323–32; with permission.)

approximately 50% would develop diabetes within 7 years. In contrast, it would take approximately 18 years for 50% of the intensive lifestyle intervention–treated participants to develop diabetes and 10 years for 50% of the metformin-treated participants to develop diabetes. Thus, compared with the placebo intervention, the lifestyle intervention delays the onset of diabetes by 11 years and the metformin intervention delays the onset of diabetes by 3 years. Over a lifetime, 83% of participants treated with the placebo intervention would develop diabetes as compared with 63% of those treated with the intensive lifestyle intervention and 75% of those treated with the metformin intervention. Thus, compared with the placebo intervention, the intensive lifestyle intervention reduces the absolute risk for developing diabetes by 20% and the metformin intervention reduces the absolute risk for developing diabetes by 8%. Because the risk of microvascular and neuropathic complications and, to a lesser degree, the macrovascular complications of diabetes occur as a function of the duration of diabetes,[17] delaying the onset and preventing the development of diabetes substantially reduce the negative effect of diabetes on the quality of life and the cost of both complications and comorbidities.

Several investigators have assessed the cost-effectiveness of lifestyle and/or medication interventions compared with that of usual care for the primary prevention of type 2 diabetes.[27–33] A prospective economic analysis conducted by the DPP Research Group estimated that the case finding cost was approximately $140 per subject randomized.[34] The lifestyle intervention for diabetes prevention cost approximately $1400 per person in the first year and approximately $700 per person per year thereafter.[34] Another analysis of a community-based lifestyle intervention program implemented through Young Men's Christian Associations found that the cost of the intervention was substantially less, approximately $300 per person per year.[35] The average wholesale price of metformin at the dose used in the DPP was approximately $300 per year.[34] The cost of acarbose as used in the STOP-NIDDM (Study to Prevent Non-Insulin-Dependent Diabetes Mellitus) Trial was approximately $1400 per person per year,[32] and the cost of rosiglitazone as used in the DREAM (Diabetes Reduction Assessment with Ramipril and Rosiglitazone Medication) trial was approximately $2000 per person per year. However, metformin is now available as a generic medication, and acarbose and thiazolidinediones will become generic. The usual cost of a generic medication is approximately 25% that of the brand medication cost.[27]

With respect to the quality of life, the DPP Research Group demonstrated that the quality of life is better with the intensive lifestyle intervention than with metformin or usual care and no different with metformin relative to usual care.[36] Clinical trials of acarbose and rosiglitazone for diabetes prevention have not included prospective utility assessments. The quality of life associated with these interventions may be no different than that associated with usual care, but it is possible that the gastrointestinal side effects associated with acarbose[10] and the weight gain associated with rosiglitazone[11] might be associated with some decrement in the quality of life.

With respect to intervention effectiveness, it is clear that the lifestyle intervention and thiazolidinediones are the most effective in preventing diabetes, with relative risk reductions of between 29% and 58% for lifestyle interventions[6–9] and between 55% and 60%[8,11] for thiazolidinediones. Metformin reduced the relative risk for development of diabetes by 26% to 31%[8,9] and acarbose by 25%.[10]

With respect to long-term health outcomes, the DPP demonstrated improved cardiovascular intermediate outcomes (blood pressure and lipids) associated with lifestyle and metformin interventions but no clear effect of these interventions on cardiovascular events (stroke, myocardial infarction) or survival.[8,37] The STOP-NIDDM study

Table 1
Cost-effectiveness of interventions for the primary prevention of type 2 diabetes

Intervention Type	Author, Year	Country	Time Horizon (y)	Cost Per Life-Year	Cost Per QALY Gained
Lifestyle	Segal et al,[28] 1998	Australia	25	Cost saving to A$2600 (US $1659; 1998)	a
	Palmer et al,[29] 2004	Australia, France, Germany, Switzerland, United Kingdom	Lifetime	Cost saving to €6400 (US $8056; 2004)	—
	Caro et al,[30] 2004	Canada	10	Can$700 (US $551; 2004)	—
	Herman,[27] 2005	United States	Lifetime	—	$1100
	Eddy et al,[31] 2005	United States	30	—	$143,000
	Icks et al,[33] 2007	Germany	3	—	€4664 (US $6269; 2007)
Metformin	Palmer et al,[29] 2004	Australia, France, Germany, Switzerland, United Kingdom	Lifetime	Costsaving to €5400 (US $6836; 2004)	—
	Caro et al,[30] 2004	Canada	10	Cost saving	$1800
	Herman,[27] 2005	United States	Lifetime	—	$35,400
	Eddy et al,[31] 2005	United States	30	—	
Acarbose	Caro et al,[30] 2004	Canada	10	Cost saving	—
	Josse et al,[32] 2006	Spain, Germany, Sweden	3	Cost saving to €800 (US $947; 2006)	—

a Results of the analysis were not reported.

showed a statistically significant effect of acarbose on the incidence of cardiovascular disease but has not reported a survival benefit.[38]

With respect to intervention safety, the DPP and the STOP-NIDDM study suggested that lifestyle intervention, metformin, and acarbose are safe.[8,10] Increased risks of heart failure[11] and fractures[39] have been associated with thiazolidinedione treatment, potentially limiting its usefulness for diabetes prevention. The safety of thiazolidinediones with respect to cardiovascular disease and survival remain controversial.[40,41]

The literature on the cost utility of diabetes prevention has recently been comprehensively reviewed.[42] Although there is no universally accepted rule to determine when an intervention is cost-effective, Laupacis and colleagues[43] have proposed a system to rate economic evaluations on the likely magnitude of the net benefit associated with the intervention. This system proposes rating interventions according to the cost per QALY gained. Current consensus is that, in the United States, interventions that cost less than $50,000 per QALY gained are an appropriate way to use resources, those that cost $50,000 to $100,000 are probably appropriate, but those that cost more than $100,000 may not represent a good value for money.

Table 1 summarizes the economic analyses that have adopted a single-payer perspective, assessed QALYs, and discounted both costs and outcomes. The costs of the treatments for the primary prevention of type 2 diabetes range from less than $1000 to approximately $20,000 per QALY gained. Of the 6 published analyses of lifestyle interventions, 4 found that lifestyle intervention was cost saving or required only a modest expenditure per life-year or QALY gained, making it extremely cost-effective. Similarly, 3 of the 4 published analyses of metformin therapy found it to be cost saving or extremely cost-effective. The 2 shorter-term analyses of acarbose for diabetes prevention demonstrated it to be cost saving or extremely cost-effective. No published studies have analyzed the cost-effectiveness of thiazolidinedione treatment for diabetes prevention.

SUMMARY

The costs associated with diabetes in the United States are enormous and growing. Although environmental and social interventions to address the underlying causative risk factors for diabetes, including obesity and physical inactivity, are promising, their effectiveness and cost-effectiveness are currently not established. Although screening and intensive lifestyle interventions and interventions with metformin and acarbose that have targeted individuals at a high risk for diabetes are more expensive than usual care, they are effective and safe. Lifestyle interventions directly improve the quality of life and delay or prevent the decrement in the quality of life and the costs associated with diabetes and its complications. Metformin and acarbose interventions are effective in delaying or preventing the decrement of the quality of life and the costs associated with diabetes and its complications. As a result, intensive lifestyle, metformin, and acarbose interventions are cost-effective. Such interventions should be adopted by health systems and widely applied to at-risk populations. Rigorous application of health economic principles to medical decision making may help to improve the value obtained for health care resources in the United States.

REFERENCES

1. Herman WH. The economics of diabetes mellitus. In: Davidson JK, editor. Clinical diabetes mellitus: a problem-oriented approach. 3rd edition. New York: Thieme; 2000. p. 815–28.

2. American Diabetes Association. Economic costs of diabetes in the U.S. in 2007. Diabetes Care 2008;31:596–615.
3. Narayan VK, Boyle JP, Thompson TJ, et al. Lifetime risk for diabetes mellitus in the United States. JAMA 2003;290:1884–90.
4. Goldman L, Cook EF. The decline in ischemic heart disease mortality rates: an analysis of the comparative effects of medical interventions and changes in lifestyles. Ann Intern Med 1984;101:825–36.
5. The HEALTHY Study Group. A school-based intervention for diabetes risk reduction. N Engl J Med 2010;363:443–53.
6. Pan XR, Li GW, Hu YH, et al. Effects of diet and exercise in preventing NIDDM in people with impaired glucose tolerance. The Da Qing IGT and Diabetes Study. Diabetes Care 1997;20:537–44.
7. Tuomilehto J, Lindstrom J, Eriksson JG, et al. Prevention of type 2 diabetes mellitus by changes in lifestyle among subjects with impaired glucose tolerance. N Engl J Med 2001;344:1343–50.
8. Knowler WC, Barrett-Connor E, Fowler SE, et al. Reduction in the incidence of type 2 diabetes with lifestyle intervention or metformin. N Engl J Med 2002;346: 393–403.
9. Ramachandran A, Snehalatha C, Mary S, et al. The Indian Diabetes Prevention Programme shows that lifestyle modification and metformin prevent type 2 diabetes in Asian Indian subjects with impaired glucose tolerance (IDPP-1). Diabetologia 2006;49:289–97.
10. Chiasson JL, Josse RG, Gomis R, et al. Acarbose for prevention of type 2 diabetes mellitus: the STOP-NIDDM randomized trial. Lancet 2002;359:2072–7.
11. Gerstein HC, Yusuf S, Bosch J, et al. Effect of rosiglitazone on the frequency of diabetes in patients with impaired glucose tolerance or impaired fasting glucose: a randomized controlled trial. Lancet 2006;368:1096–105.
12. Nichols GA, Glauber HS, Brown JB. Type 2 diabetes: incremental medical care costs during the 8 years preceding diagnosis. Diabetes Care 2000;23:1654–9.
13. Nichols GA, Arondekar B, Herman WH. Medical care costs one year after identification of hyperglycemia below the threshold for diabetes. Med Care 2008;46: 287–92.
14. Nichols GA, Arondekar B, Herman WH. Complications of dysglycemia and medical costs associated with nondiabetic hyperglycemia. Am J Manag Care 2008;14:791–8.
15. Brown JB, Pedula KL, Bakst AW. The progressive cost of complications in type 2 diabetes mellitus. Arch Intern Med 1999;159:1873–80.
16. Brandle M, Zhou H, Smith BR, et al. The direct medical cost of type 2 diabetes mellitus. Diabetes Care 2003;26:2300–4.
17. Caro JJ, Ward AJ, O'Brien JA. Lifetime costs of complications resulting from type 2 diabetes in the U.S. Diabetes Care 2002;25:476–81.
18. Anandacoomarasamy A, Caterson ID, Leibman S, et al. Influence of BMI on health-related quality of life: comparison between an obese adult cohort and age-matched population norms. Obesity (Silver Spring) 2009;17:2114–8.
19. Sach TH, Barton GR, Doherty M, et al. The relationship between body mass index and health-related quality of life: comparing the EQ-5D, EuroQol VAS and SF-6D. Int J Obes 2007;31:189–96.
20. Lee AJ, Morgan CL, Morrissey M, et al. Evaluation of the association between the EQ-5D$_{index}$ (health-related utility) and body mass index (obesity) in hospital-treated people with type 1 diabetes, type 2 diabetes and with no diagnosed diabetes. Diabet Med 2005;22:1482–6.

21. U.K. Prospective Diabetes Study Group: quality of life in type 2 diabetic patients is affected by complications but not by intensive policies to improve blood glucose or blood pressure control (UKPDS 37). Diabetes Care 1999;22: 1125–36.

22. Redekop WK, Koopmanschap MA, Stolk RP, et al. Health-related quality of life and treatment satisfaction in Dutch patients with type 2 diabetes. Diabetes Care 2002;25:458–63.

23. Ragnarson Tennvall G, Apelqvist J. Health-related quality of life in patients with diabetes mellitus and foot ulcers. J Diabetes Complications 2000;14:235–41.

24. Glasziou P, Alexander J, Beller E, et al, ADVANCE Collaborative Group. Which health-related quality of life score? A comparison of alternative utility measures in patients with type 2 diabetes in the ADVANCE trial. Heath Qual Life Outcomes 2007;5:21–31.

25. Coffey JT, Brandle M, Zhou H, et al. Valuing health-related quality of life in diabetes. Diabetes Care 2002;25:2238–43.

26. Herman WH. Economic analyses of diabetes interventions: rationale, principles, findings, and interpretation. Endocrinologist 1999;9:113–7.

27. Herman WH, Hoerger TJ, Brandle M, et al. The cost-effectiveness of lifestyle modification or metformin in preventing type 2 diabetes in adults with impaired glucose tolerance. Ann Intern Med 2005;142:323–32.

28. Segal L, Dalton AC, Richardson J. Cost-effectiveness of the primary prevention of non-insulin dependent diabetes mellitus. Health Promot Int 1998;13:197–209.

29. Palmer AJ, Roze S, Valentine WJ, et al. Intensive lifestyle changes or metformin in patients with impaired glucose tolerance: modeling the long-term health economic implications of the diabetes prevention program in Australia, France, Germany, Switzerland, and the United Kingdom. Clin Ther 2004;26:304–21.

30. Caro JJ, Getsios D, Caro I, et al. Economic evaluation of therapeutic interventions to prevent type 2 diabetes in Canada. Diabet Med 2004;21:1229–36.

31. Eddy DM, Schlessinger L, Kahn R. Clinical outcomes and cost-effectiveness of strategies for managing people at high risk for diabetes. Ann Intern Med 2005; 143:251–64.

32. Josse RG, McGuire AJ, Saal GB. A review of the economic evidence for acarbose in the prevention of diabetes and cardiovascular events in individuals with impaired glucose tolerance. Int J Clin Pract 2006;60:847–55.

33. Icks A, Rathmann W, Haastert B, et al, on behalf of the KORA Study Group. Clinical and cost-effectiveness of primary prevention of type 2 diabetes in a 'real world' routine healthcare setting: model based on the KORA Survey 2000. Diabet Med 2007;24:473–80.

34. Herman WH, Brandle M, Zhang P, et al, The Diabetes Prevention Program Research Group. Costs associated with the primary prevention of type 2 diabetes mellitus in the Diabetes Prevention Program. Diabetes Care 2003;26:36–47.

35. Ackermann RT, Marrero DG. Adapting the Diabetes Prevention Program lifestyle intervention for delivery in the community. The YMCA Model. Diabetes Educ 2007;33:69–78.

36. Herman WH, Brandle M, Zhang P, et al, The Diabetes Prevention Program Research Group. Within-trial cost-effectiveness of lifestyle intervention or metformin for the primary prevention of type 2 diabetes. Diabetes Care 2003;26: 2518–23.

37. Diabetes Prevention Program Research Group. 10-year follow-up of diabetes incidence and weight loss in the Diabetes Prevention Program Outcomes Study. Lancet 2009;374:1677–86.

38. Chiasson JL, Josse RG, Gomis R, et al, STOP-NIDDM Trial Research Group. Acarbose treatment and the risk of cardiovascular disease and hypertension in patients with impaired glucose tolerance: the STOP-NIDDM trial. JAMA 2003; 290:486–94.
39. Kahn SE, Haffner SM, Heise MA, et al, ADOPT Study Group. Glycemic durability of rosiglitazone, metformin, or glyburide monotherapy. N Engl J Med 2006;355: 2427–43.
40. Graham DJ, Oeullet-Hellstrom R, MaCurdy TE, et al. Risk of acute myocardial infarction, stroke, heart failure, and death in elderly Medicare patients treated with rosiglitazone or pioglitazone. JAMA 2010;304:411–8.
41. Wertz DA, Chang CL, Sarawate CA, et al. Risk of cardiovascular events and all-cause mortality in patients treated with thiazolidinediones in a managed-care population. Circ Cardiovasc Qual Outcomes 2010;3:538–45.
42. Li R, Zhang P, Barker LE, et al. Cost-effectiveness of interventions to prevent and control diabetes mellitus: a systematic review. Diabetes Care 2010;33:1872–94.
43. Laupacis A, Feeny D, Detsky AS, et al. How attractive does a new technology have to be to warrant adoption and utilization? Tentative guidelines for using clinical and economic evaluations. Can Med Assoc J 1992;146:473–81.

Treatment Recommendations for Prediabetes

Robert E. Ratner, MD[a,b,*], Anpalakan Sathasivam, MD[c]

KEYWORDS

• Prediabetes • Diabetes • Metformin • Lifestyle intervention

A variety of definitions and diagnostic cutpoints have been promulgated for predia-betes over the past 5 years, without universal agreement. International professional organizations agree, however, that current scientific evidence justifies the intervention in high-risk individuals and populations for the delay or prevention of progression to diabetes. With many clinical trials examining the efficacy of prevention strategies, life-style intervention with the goals of decreasing caloric intake, increasing exercise to at least 150 minutes weekly, and losing 5% to 7% of body weight is universally accepted as the primary intervention strategy. Secondary intervention with a variety of pharma-cologic therapies (predominantly metformin) is advocated in very high-risk individuals or in the absence of a clinical response to lifestyle modification. Surgical intervention is currently recognized as beneficial, but with limited enthusiasm.

DIAGNOSIS OF PREDIABETES AND DIABETES

Much has been written in the past 3 years on the continuous relationship between glucose and micro- and macrovascular complications of diabetes mellitus. In this issue of the *Medical Clinics of North America*, chapters by Buysschaert and Bergman, and Shaw have provided reviews of the current definitions and diagnostic criteria for prediabetes and diabetes. Although this article does not reiterate their reviews, it is imperative to understand that these are somewhat arbitrary categorical cutoffs for disease based on assessments of disease risk, metabolic complications, and popula-tion distributions of plasma glucose.[1] Thresholds for increasing risk of retinopathy serve as the primary cutoff for defining diabetes by fasting plasma glucose (FPG), oral glucose tolerance test (OGTT), and hemoglobin A1c (HbA1c).[2,3] There remains

[a] MedStar Health Research Institute, 6525 Belcrest Road, Suite 700, Hyattsville, MD, 20782, USA
[b] Division of Endocrinology, Georgetown University School of Medicine, 4000 Reservoir Road NW, Building D Second Floor, Washington, DC, USA
[c] Division of Endocrinology, Georgetown University School of Medicine, 4000 Reservoir Road NW, Building D Second Floor, Washington, DC 20007, USA
* Corresponding author. MedStar Health Research Institute, 6525 Belcrest Road, Suite 700, Hyattsville, MD 20782.
E-mail address: Robert.Ratner@medstar.net

Med Clin N Am 95 (2011) 385–395
doi:10.1016/j.mcna.2010.11.007
0025-7125/11/$ – see front matter © 2011 Elsevier Inc. All rights reserved.

medical.theclinics.com

much controversy, however, because complications can be seen even earlier than with the accepted diagnostic cutoffs. In the Diabetes Prevention Program (DPP), 7.9% of impaired glucose tolerance (IGT) subjects had documented diabetic retinopathy, whereas12.6% of the subjects with newly diagnosed diabetes had prevalent retinopathy.[4] A recent review documents the broad development of classic diabetic retinopathy in those individuals before the diagnosis of diabetes.[5] This should not be surprising, because the Hyperglycemia and Adverse Pregnancy Outcome Study also demonstrated the continuous relationship between maternal glucose concentrations at levels below that diagnostic of diabetes and the adverse pregnancy outcomes of both excess birth weight and cord blood C-peptide concentration above the 90th percentile, representing fetal hyperinsulinemia.[6] Given that cardiovascular disease (CVD) is the primary cause of morbidity and mortality in those patients with either prediabetes or diabetes, the observation of a linear relationship between 2-hour post-challenge glucose levels—starting well below the threshold for the diagnosis of diabetes—and cardiovascular events further obscures the proposed categorical cutoff for diagnosis and treatment of diabetes.[7]

Recognizing this continuous relationship between glycemia and risk of diabetes and its complications, the 2010 American Diabetes Association (ADA) guidelines now more formally refer to impaired fasting glucose (IFG) and IGT as "categories of increased risk of diabetes" with risks extending continuously even beyond the defined categories.[8] This article suggests that following glucose as a continuous variable with interventions recommended on the basis of risk of metabolic progression and the development of complications is a more logical clinical approach.[9] The potential interventions for the treatment of prediabetes and categories of increased risk of diabetes are reviewed.

CURRENT RECOMMENDATIONS FOR SCREENING FOR PREDIABETES

Screening for the DPP was based on an analysis of 6 prospective epidemiologic studies revealing a significantly increased risk of incident diabetes (57 per 1000 person-years) in those with IGT by standard ADA criteria.[10] Subsequently, the DPP demonstrated an 11% per year incidence of diabetes in its enrollees with IGT and an increased fasting glucose.[11] These incident rates of diabetes pale in comparison to the almost 50% 5-year risk of diabetes encountered by women with a history of gestational diabetes mellitus (GDM).[12] Despite these remarkable observations, the U.S. Preventive Services Task Force (USPSTF) recommends screening for prediabetes only for those adults with blood pressure greater than 135/80 mm Hg whether or not treated.[13]

The implications of missing individuals at increased risk of diabetes are unknown, but the cost-effectiveness of screening has been examined (see the article by William H. Herman elsewhere in this issue for further exploration of this topic). Three analyses examined the cost-effectiveness of screening specifically. The Centers for Disease Control and Prevention analysis provides a range of $247 to $332 per case of prediabetes and unrecognized diabetes diagnosed.[14] The DPP cost-effectiveness analysis reports a robust $8181 per quality-adjusted life-year gained in screening and subsequently treating prediabetes.[15] More recently, Kahn and colleagues[16] used the Archimedes model to examine strategies in which screening is done opportunistically in combination with blood pressure measurement and lipid testing and showed that this approach has the lowest cost per quality-adjusted life-year gained.

Currently, several professional organizations have weighed in regarding screening and treatment recommendations for prediabetes. **Box 1** summarizes the published screening recommendations from these societies. All go well beyond the

---

Box 1
Published guidelines for screening for prediabetes

ADA[8,17,18]: Screening should be done in all adults who are overweight (body mass index [BMI] $\geq$25 kg/m^2) and have other risk factors. In adults with normal weight and without any risk factors, screening must begin at age 45. Fasting plasma glucose (FPG), HbA1c, or OGTT can be used for the screening purpose. If the screening test is normal, then screening should be repeated every 3 years.

The Endocrine Society[19]: Screen patients for components of metabolic syndrome, as defined by the American Heart Association/National Heart, Lung, and Blood Institute, for at least every 3 years; at least 3 components in any patient puts him/her for high risk for metabolic syndrome. Patients with previous history of diabetes should be screened for diabetes every 1 to 2 years using FPG or OGTT. All patients with metabolic risk should undergo global risk assessment for 10-year risk for coronary heart disease or cerebral vascular disease using Framingham and Prospective Cardiovascular Münster (PROCAM) scoring or The European Systematic Coronary Risk Evaluation algorithm before starting preventive therapy.

American Association of Clinical Endocrinologists (AACE)[20,21]: Subjects with high-risk factors for developing diabetes should be screened using the 2-hour OGTT or FPG to establish the diagnosis of prediabetes.

International Diabetes Federation (IDF)[22]: Identification of the high-risk group based on central obesity, family history of diabetes, age, cardiovascular history, history of GDM, and use of drugs that predispose to diabetes. Use of FPG to screen and if plasma glucose is 110 to 125 range then use an OGTT; measurement of other risk factors, including waist circumference, blood pressure, family history of diabetes, raised triglyceride, and pre-existing CVD.

Indian Health Service (IHS)[23]: Use FPG or 2-hour OGTT to screen high-risk patients.

Canadian Diabetes Association (CDA)[24]: Every 3 years, all subjects 40 years of age and older should be screened for type 2 diabetes mellitus using FPG. Subjects with risk factors for type 2 diabetes mellitus should be screened earlier using FPG or OGTT. Subjects with FPG should be screened using OGTT to identify those with IGT or diabetes mellitus.

Australian Diabetes Society (ADS)[25]: Adults who are overweight should be screened for prediabetes/diabetes using FPG, and subjects with FPG greater than or equal to 100 mg/dL should be screened for IGT/diabetes mellitus by using OGTT.

---

recommendations of the USPSTF recommendation to include evaluation of obesity and other risk factors, including family history, in the decision to screen. Most agree that high-risk individuals should have repeat screening at least every 3 years. Screening, however, is important only if interventions are available to alter the natural history of the underlying disease. The recommendations for screening are all predicated on the subsequent initiation of interventions proved in controlled clinical trials (see the article by Ramachandran elsewhere in this issue for further exploration of this topic) to decrease progression to diabetes. The remainder of this article examines the various national, international, and professional society recommendations for the treatment of prediabetes.

INTERVENTIONS SHOWN TO REDUCE CONVERSION FROM PREDIABETES TO DIABETES
Lifestyle Modification

The relationship among obesity and the development of diabetes led to the delineation of the pathophysiologic relationships of obesity (predominantly central or visceral adiposity), insulin resistance, beta-cell decompensation, and the ultimate rise in FPG and postchallenge glucose levels, which have come to be defined as prediabetes and diabetes.[26] Lifestyle modification with mild to moderate calorie reduction with or without exercise demonstrates the most consistent and reproducible reduction in diabetes progression. The Da Qing Study[27] randomized communities to diet-only, exercise-only, or diet-plus-exercise, with an associated relative risk reduction in new-onset diabetes of 31%, 46%, and 42%, respectively. Perhaps most interesting was the 20-year follow-up of this population demonstrating a sustained 51% relative risk reduction in the development of diabetes for the combined diet and exercise group.[28] Although no difference was observed in first CVD events, a trend in reduced CVD mortality (27% relative risk reduction) and all-cause mortality (10% relative risk reduction) was found.

Both the Finnish Diabetes Prevention Study and the US DPP confirmed the beneficial impact of lifestyle modification in more rigorous individual randomized controlled trials.[10,29] Despite different approaches to lifestyle modification, both studies strove to achieve a 7% reduction in body weight. Although initially achieved, this degree of weight loss could not be sustained, with the DPP ending with a 4% weight loss at study end. Regardless of the weight regain, both studies reported a 58% reduction in incident diabetes. The Finnish Diabetes Prevention Study cohort were more successful than the DPP cohort in maintaining weight loss after the initial intervention of the clinical trials, but both studies preserve the diabetes conversion benefit over the long term.[30,31] Together with the Indian Diabetes Prevention Program (IDPP),[32] these studies provide robust and reproducible evidence of the efficacy and generalizability of lifestyle modification in different age, ethnic, and socioeconomic populations.

Metformin

Metformin, a biguanide that reduces hepatic glucose production and causes mild weight loss, has been studied in both the DPP[10] and IDPP.[32] The DPP, using a recommended dose of 850 mg twice a day, noted a 31% reduction in diabetes conversion compared with placebo in the core study. Detailed predefined analysis of the DPP database showed metformin effective in preventing diabetes, particularly in younger individuals, those with a BMI greater than 35, and women with a history of GDM.[33] In general, metformin was well tolerated, although 29% failed to take greater than or equal to 80% of their medication over time.[34] After a limited washout, the metformin effect was reduced to 25%.[35] In the DPP Outcomes Study, the mild weight loss associated with metformin therapy was maintained at 10 years' follow-up and there was a persistent 18% reduction in progression to diabetes compared with placebo.[31] The IDPP used a lower metformin dose (250 mg twice a day) and noted a 26% reduction in incident diabetes. This study also included a combined lifestyle plus metformin arm, which failed to demonstrate any additive effect of the combination.[32]

Thiazolidinediones

Three different peroxisome proliferator-activated receptor-γ agonists of the thiazolidinedione class have been studied in the setting of diabetes prevention. This class of drugs improves insulin sensitivity, despite causing weight gain. Troglitazone, removed from the market due to its association with liver toxicity, was used in the DPP[35,36] as well as in the Troglitazone in the Prevention of Diabetes (TRIPOD) study of women with a history of GDM.[37] Pioglitazone was used as continuing therapy after TRIPOD[38] as well as used in the Actos Now for the Prevention of Diabetes Trial (ACTNOW Trial).[39] Rosiglitazone was examined in the Diabetes Reduction Assessment with Ramipril and Rosiglitazone Medication (DREAM) trial in a factorial design with ramipril, an angiotensin-converting enzyme inhibitor[40] as well as in combination with metformin in the Canadian Normoglycemia Outcomes Evaluation Trial.[41] Despite a highly significant reduction in diabetes incidence, as high as 78%, the side-effect profile, including the aforementioned liver abnormalities with troglitazone, bone fractures, congestive heart failure, and cost, limit recommending this class for first-line use in diabetes prevention.

Enteric Enzyme Inhibitors

Inhibition of both α-glucosidase and lipase has been studied in the setting of prediabetes, examining the impact of relative malabsorption on diabetes incidence. Acarbose, an α-glucosidase inhibitor, not only reduced the incidence of diabetes by 25% in the Study to Prevent Noninsulin-Dependent Diabetes Mellitus (STOP-NIDDM)[42] but also suggested a positive impact on the development of CVD events.[43] The acarbose treatment arm was associated with a high discontinuation rate due to gastrointestinal intolerance, complicating the interpretation of the STOP-NIDDM. The therapy is limited by gastrointestinal side effects and the loss of efficacy after short-term discontinuation of therapy. Orlistat blocks fat absorption, resulting in weight loss either through steatorrhea or through behavior modification of eating behavior. In the Xenical in the Prevention of Diabetes in Obese Subjects Study,[44] orlistat reduced diabetes incidence by 37% but was severely limited by gastrointestinal side effects.

Surgical Approaches

Bariatric surgical approaches intend to affect weight loss by limiting calorie intake via mechanical obstruction or by impairing nutrient absorption through intestinal bypass. Significant weight loss is seen in most subjects able to tolerate the procedures. Bypass procedures also result in significant incretin hormone changes with remarkable increases in glucagon-like peptide 1 well before weight loss occurs. Early reports of gastric bypass surgery reported reversion to normal glucose tolerance in 78% of individuals with diabetes and 98% of those with IGT.[45] In a subsequent controlled trial, the Swedish Obese Subjects study[46] surgical intervention produced a 75% relative risk reduction of diabetes compared with medical controls over a 10-year period. The morbidity, complexity, and cost are the primary limiting factors of this approach.

COST-EFFECTIVENESS CONSIDERATIONS IN THE TREATMENT OF PREDIABETES

Clinical trial data provide evidence of efficacy of a particular intervention, and the approaches (discussed previously) demonstrate the degree of diabetes prevention independent of cost or potential harms. Treatment guidelines, alternatively, incorporate efficacy of an intervention, potential treatment acceptability and adherence, side effects, and cost. Cost-effectiveness analysis can aid in the determination of which therapies should be recommended for a particular indication based on their projected usefulness (see the article by William H. Herman elsewhere in this issue for review of the economic impact of diabetes prevention). Ultimately, the decision to screen for prediabetes and initiate therapy to prevent or delay the progression to diabetes is made in the expectation that morbidities associated with the disease can be reduced and quality of life of individuals improved at a cost that is reasonable to payors and society. Detailed cost-effectiveness analysis has been undertaken for the DPP within the study[47,48] as well as in computer projections of the life of participants.[49] Although some disagreement exists about the assumptions used in the computer modeling,[50] DPP projections show clear cost-effectiveness for both lifestyle and metformin interventions for the delay or prevention of diabetes. Clinical data together with these cost-effectiveness analyses feed into the consideration of practice guidelines.[51]

TREATMENT RECOMMENDATIONS

Published guidelines on the approach to patients with prediabetes include a consensus statement from the ADA, the IHS guidelines for care of the adults with prediabetes and/or metabolic syndrome, and a position statement from the ADS and the Australian Diabetes Educators Association (**Table 1**). The recommendations

Table 1
Key features of selected published recommendations on prediabetes

	ADA Consensus Statement (2007)[17]	Indian Health Services Guidelines for Care of Adults with Prediabetes and/or the Metabolic Syndrome in Clinical Settings (2006)[23]	Australian Diabetes Society and Australian Diabetes Educators Association Position Statement (2007)[25]
IFG	FPG >100 mg/dL (5.6 mmol/L) but <126 mg/dL (7.0 mmol/L) and 2-h plasma glucose <200 mg/dL (11.1 mmol/L)	FPG >100 mg/dL (5.6 mmol/L) but <126 mg/dL (7.0 mmol/L)	FPG >110 mg/dL (6.1 mmol/L) and <126 mg/dL (7.0 mmol/L) with 2-h plasma glucose <140 mg/dL (7.8 mmol/L)
IGT	FPG <126 mg/dL (7.0 mmol/L) and 2-h plasma glucose >140 mg/dL (7.8 mmol/L) but <200 mg/dL (11.1 mmol/L)	2-h plasma glucose >140 mg/dL (7.8 mmol/L) but <200 mg/dL (11.1 mmol/L)	FPG <126 mg/dL (7.0 mmol/L) and 2-h plasma glucose >140 mg/dL (7.8 mmol/L) but <200 mg/dL (11.1 mmol/L)
Who should be screened for prediabetes?	Individuals with risk factors for diabetes should be screened for prediabetes	Annual testing of individuals at risk for developing diabetes	Incidental detection when screening for diabetes
Method of screening	FPG; 2-h OGTT if metformin therapy is considered	FPG; Optional 2-h OGTT if resources permit	Incidental detection when screening for diabetes
Recommended treatment	Lifestyle modification for IFG or IGT; Lifestyle modification and/or metformin for IFG and IGT and at least one of the following: age <60 y, BMI >35 kg/m², family history of diabetes in first-degree relatives, elevated triglycerides, reduced HDL-C, hypertension, HbA1c >6.0%	Lifestyle changes; Consideration of metformin on an individualized basis; depression screening and cardiovascular risk reduction also recommended	Intensive lifestyle intervention for a minimum of 6 months before consideration of pharmacotherapy
Follow-up	Metformin treatment: semiannual HbA1c; Lifestyle intervention: annual follow-up	Monitor glucose values every 6 months	75-g OGTT, initially performed annually, then individualized retesting every 1–3 y

Data from American Diabetes Association. 2010 Standards of medical care in diabetes. Diabetes Care 2010;33(Suppl 1):S11–61.

on treatment of prediabetes differ slightly. Both The Endocrine Society[19] and the AACE[20,21] recommend lifestyle intervention preferentially over pharmacologic therapy. The ADA consensus statement stratifies therapy based on whether or not patients have isolated IFG, isolated IGT, or a combination of IFG and IGT, allowing for consideration in differences in the underlying physiology and disease progression.[17] The most recent standards of care, however, focus more on A1c and associated risk factors.[8] Lifestyle modification with a weight loss goal of 5% to 10% is recommended along with 30 minutes of moderate daily physical activity.

Recommendations for the use of metformin are tailored toward individuals who may have greater benefit from this drug observed in the DPP and for those at greater risk of progression to diabetes. Thus, metformin is considered for individuals less than 60 years of age, individuals with a BMI of at least 35 kg/m^2, and those at increased risk, such as having a family history of diabetes in first-degree relatives, elevated triglycerides, reduced high-density-lipoprotein cholesterol (HDL-C), hypertension, or HbA1c greater than 6.0%.[17] Additionally, metformin seemed equally effective as lifestyle in those women with a history of GDM.[33] The IHS guidelines similarly advocate lifestyle changes with consideration for metformin or pioglitazone on an individualized basis.[23] The Australian guidelines recommend lifestyle intervention as first-line therapy for a minimum of 6 months before consideration of pharmacotherapy,[25] whereas the CDA considers the use of either metformin, an α-glucosidase inhibitor, or a thiazolidinedione in those with no known CVD.[24] The IDF reserves pharmacologic therapy for those unable to achieve the goals of lifestyle modification and recommends metformin, acarbose, and orlistat but not thiazolidinediones due to the potential for weight gain and congestive heart failure associated with this class as therapeutic options.[22]

The decision to initiate therapy for prediabetes should be undertaken with the full understanding of provider and patient that any therapy requires a long-term commitment. Ongoing monitoring of metabolic status and potential therapeutic side effects are required with treatment modification undertaken if goals are not achieved or intolerable side effects are encountered. Efficacy data now provide several proved avenues for both providers and patients to pursue in the treatment of prediabetes, so therapies can be individualized to patient acceptance and tolerance. Virtually all professional societies recommend lifestyle modification as initial intervention with consideration of pharmacologic and surgical therapy reserved for those at highest risk or demonstrating progressive glycemic deterioration. The demonstration that intervention positively affects the natural history of diabetes and its complications is

---

Box 2
Summary of guideline recommendations for the treatment of prediabetes

Lifestyle modification/weight loss: recommended by ADA, The Endocrine Society, AACE, IHS, American Academy of Pediatrics, CDA, ADS, and IDF

Metformin: recommended on an individual basis by ADA, IHS, CDA, ADS, and IDF

Thiazolidinediones: considered on an individual basis by IHS, CDA, and ADS

α-Glucosidase inhibitors: considered on an individual basis by CDA, ADS, and IDF

Orlisat: considered on an individual basis by ADS and IDF

Bariatric surgery: considered on an individual basis by IHS

Phentermine, sibutramine, or rimonabant: not recommended by any of the above organizations.

suggested by computer modeling,[49] but continued observation of cohorts previously enrolled in controlled clinical trials is necessary to prove ultimately that early intervention benefits both individuals and society (**Box 2**).

REFERENCES

1. World Health Organization/International Diabetes Federation 2006 Definition and Diagnosis of Diabetes Mellitus and Intermediate Hyperglycemia: report of a WHO/IDF consultation. Available at: http://www.who.int/diabetes/publications/Definition%20and%20diagnosis%20of%20diabetes_new.pdf. Accessed April 28, 2008.
2. The Expert Committee on the Diagnosis and Classification of Diabetes Mellitus Report of the expert committee on the diagnosis and classification of diabetes mellitus. Diabetes Care 1997;20:785–91.
3. Ito C, Maeda R, Ishida S, et al. Importance of OGTT for diagnosing diabetes mellitus based on prevalence and incidence of retinopathy. Diabetes Res Clin Pract 2000;49:181–6.
4. Diabetes Prevention Program Research Group. The prevalence of retinopathy in impaired glucose tolerance and recent-onset diabetes in the Diabetes Prevention Program. Diabet Med 2007;24:137–44.
5. Nguyen TT, Wang JJ, Wong TY. Retinal vascular changes in pre-diabetes and prehypertension. Diabetes Care 2007;30:2708–15.
6. The HAPO Study Cooperative Research Group. Hyperglycemia and adverse pregnancy outcomes. N Engl J Med 2008;358:1991–2002.
7. DECODE Study Group, European Diabetes Epidemiology Group. Is the current definition for diabetes relevant to mortality risk from all causes and cardiovascular and noncardiovascular diseases? Diabetes Care 2003;26:688–96.
8. American Diabetes Association. 2010 Standards of medical care in diabetes. Diabetes Care 2010;33(Suppl 1):S11–61.
9. Aroda V, Ratner R. Approach to the patient with pre-diabetes. J Clin Endocrinol Metab 2008;93:3259–65.
10. Edelstein SL, Knowler WC, Bain RP, et al. Predictors of progression from impaired glucose tolerance to NIDDM: an analysis of six prospective studies. Diabetes 1997;46:701–10.
11. Knowler WC, Barrett-Connor E, Fowler SE, et al. Diabetes Prevention Program Research Group. Reduction in the incidence of type 2 diabetes with lifestyle intervention or metformin. N Engl J Med 2002;346:393–403.
12. Kim C, Newton KM, Knopp RH. Gestational diabetes mellitus and the incidence of type 2 diabetes. Diabetes Care 2002;25:1862–8.
13. U.S. Preventive Services Task Force. Screening for type 2 diabetes mellitus in adults: U.S. Preventive Services Task Force recommendation statement. Ann Intern Med 2008;148:846–54.
14. Zhang P, Engelgau M, Valdez R, et al. Costs of screening for pre-diabetes among U.S. Adults. Diabetes Care 2003;26:2536–42.
15. Hoerger TJ, Hicks KA, Sorenson SW, et al. The cost-effectiveness of screening for pre-diabetes among overweight and obese U.S. adults. Diabetes Care 2007;30:2874–9.
16. Kahn R, Alperin P, Eddy D, et al. Age at initiation and frequency of screening to detect type 2 diabetes: a cost-effectiveness analysis. Lancet 2010;375(9723):1365–74.

17. Nathan DM, Davidson MB, DeFronzo RA, et al. Impaired fasting glucose and impaired glucose tolerance. Diabetes Care 2007;30:753–9.
18. American Diabetes Association, National Institute of Diabetes and Digestive and Kidney Disease. Position statement. Prevention or delay of type 2 diabetes. Diabetes Care 2004;27(Suppl 1):s47.
19. Rosenzweig JL, Ferrannini E, Grundy SM, et al. Primary prevention of cardiovascular disease and type 2 diabetes in patients at metabolic risk: an endocrine society clinical practice guideline. J Clin Endocrinol Metab 2008;93:3671–89.
20. Rodbard HW, Blonde L, Braithwaite SS, et al, AACE Diabetes Mellitus Clinical Practice Guidelines Task Force. American Association of Clinical Endocrinologists medical guidelines for clinical practice for the management of diabetes mellitus. Endocr Pract 2007;13(Suppl 1):1–68.
21. Garber AJ, Handelsman Y, Einhorn D, et al. Diagnosis and management of prediabetes in the continuum of hyperglycemia: when do the risks of diabetes begin? A consensus statement from the American College of Endocrinology and the American Association of Clinical Endocrinologists. Endocr Pract 2008; 14(7):933–46.
22. Alberti KG, Zimmet P, Shaw J. International diabetes federation: a consensus on Type 2 diabetes prevention. Diabet Med 2007;24:451–63.
23. Indian Health Service. Guidelines for care of adults with pre-diabetes and/or the metabolic syndrome in clinical settings. 2008. Available at: http://www.ihs.gov/MedicalPrograms/Diabetes/HomeDocs/Tools/ClinicalGuidelines/PreDiabetes_Guidelines_0209.pdf. Accessed April 28, 2008.
24. Canadian Diabetes Association Clinical Practice Guidelines Expert Committee. Canadian Diabetes Association for the prevention and management of diabetes in Canada. Can J Diabetes 2008;32(Suppl 1):S17–9.
25. Twigg SM, Kamp MC, Davis TM, for the Australian Diabetes Society; Australian Diabetes Educators Association, et al. Pre-diabetes: a position statement from the Australian Diabetes Society and Australian Diabetes Educators Association. Med J Aust 2007;186:461–5.
26. DeFronzo RA. Banting Lecture. From the triumvirate to the ominous octet: a new paradigm for the treatment of type 2 diabetes mellitus. Diabetes 2009;58:773–95.
27. Pan XR, Li GW, Hu YH, et al. Effects of diet and exercise in preventing NIDDM in people with impaired glucose tolerance. The Da Qing IGT and Diabetes Study. Diabetes Care 1997;20:537–44.
28. Li G, Zhang P, Wang J, et al. The long-term effect of lifestyle interventions to prevent diabetes in the China Da Qing Prevention Study: a 20 year follow-up study. Lancet 2008;371:1783–9.
29. Tuomilehto J, Lindström J, Eriksson JG, et al, Finnish Diabetes Prevention Study Group. Prevention of type 2 diabetes mellitus by changes in lifestyle among subjects with impaired glucose tolerance. N Engl J Med 2001;344:1343–50.
30. Lindstrom J, Ilanne-Parikka P, Peltonen M, et al. Sustained reduction in the incidence of type 2 diabetes by lifestyle intervention: follow-up of the Finnish Diabetes Prevention Study. Lancet 2006;368:1673–9.
31. Diabetes Prevention Program Research Group. 10-Year follow-up of diabetes incidence and weight loss in the Diabetes Prevention Program Outcomes Study. Lancet 2009;374:1677–86.
32. Ramachandran A, Snehalatha C, Mary S, et al, Vijay V for the Indian Diabetes Prevention Programme (IDPP. The Indian Diabetes Prevention Programme shows that lifestyle modification and metformin prevent type 2 diabetes in Asian Indian subjects with impaired glucose tolerance (IDPP-1). Diabetologia 2006;49:289–97.

33. Ratner RE, Christophi C, Metzger BE, et al. Prevention of diabetes in women with a history of gestational diabetes: effects of metformin and lifestyle intervention. J Clin Endocrinol Metab 2008;93:4774–9.
34. Walker EA, Molitch M, Kramer MK, et al. Adherence to preventive medications: predictors and outcomes in the Diabetes Prevention Program. Diabetes Care 2006;29:1997–2002.
35. Diabetes Prevention Program Research Group. Effects of withdrawal from metformin on the development of diabetes in the Diabetes Prevention Program. Diabetes Care 2003;26:977–80.
36. Diabetes prevention Program Research Group. Prevention of type 2 diabetes with troglitazone in the Diabetes Prevention Program. Diabetes 2005;54:1150–6.
37. Buchanan TA, Xiang AH, Peters RK, et al. Preservation of pancreatic beta-cell function and prevention of type 2 diabetes by pharmacological treatment of insulin resistance in high-risk Hispanic women. Diabetes 2002;51:2796–803.
38. Xiang AH, Peters RK, Kjos SL, et al. Effect of pioglitazone on pancreatic beta-cell function and diabetes risk in Hispanic women with prior gestational diabetes. Diabetes 2006;55:517–22.
39. Defronzo RA, Banerji M, Bray GA, et al. Actos Now for the prevention of diabetes (ACT NOW) study. BMC Endocr Disord 2009;29:9–17.
40. DREAM (Diabetes REduction Assessment with ramipril and rosiglitazone Medication) Trial Investigators, Gerstein HC, Yusuf S, et al. Effect of rosiglitazone on the frequency of diabetes in patients with impaired glucose tolerance or impaired fasting glucose: a randomised controlled trial. Lancet 2006;368:1096–105.
41. Zinman B, Harris SB, Neuman J, et al. Low-dose combination therapy with rosiglitazone and metformin to prevent type 2 diabetes mellitus (Canoe Trial): a double-blind randomized controlled trial. Lancet 2010;376:103–11.
42. Chiasson JL, Josse RG, Gomis R, et al, STOP-NIDDM Trail Research Group. Acarbose for prevention of type 2 diabetes mellitus: the STOP-NIDDM randomised trial. Lancet 2002;359:2072–7.
43. Chiasson JL, Josse RG, Gomis R, et al, STOP-NIDDM Trail Research Group. Acarbose treatment and the risk of cardiovascular disease and hypertension in patients with impaired glucose tolerance: the STOP NIDDM trial. JAMA 2003; 290:486–94.
44. Torgerson JS, Hauptman J, Boldrin MN, et al. Xenical in the prevention of Diabetes in Obese Subjects (XENDOS) study: a randomized study of orlistat as an adjunct to lifestyle changes for the prevention of type 2 diabetes in obese patients. Diabetes Care 2004;27:155–61.
45. Pories WJ, MacDonald KG Jr, Flickinger EG, et al. Is type II diabetes mellitus (NIDDM) a surgical disease? Ann Surg 1992;215:633–42.
46. Sjöström L, Lindroos AK, Peltonen M, et al, Swedish Obese Subjects Study Scientific Group. Lifestyle, diabetes, and cardiovascular risk factors 10 years after bariatric surgery. N Engl J Med 2004;351:2683–93.
47. The Diabetes Prevention Program Research Group. Costs associated with the primary prevention of type 2 diabetes mellitus in the Diabetes Prevention Program. Diabetes Care 2003;26:36–47.
48. The Diabetes Prevention Program Research Group. Within trial cost-effectiveness of lifestyle intervention or metformin for the primary prevention of type 2 diabetes. Diabetes Care 2003;26:2518–23.
49. Herman WH, Hoerger TJ, Brandle M, et al. The lifetime cost-utility of lifestyle intervention or Metformin for the primary prevention of type 2 diabetes mellitus. Ann Intern Med 2005;142:323–32.

50. Engelgau MM. Trying to predict the future for people with diabetes: a tough but important task. Ann Intern Med 2005;143:301–2.

51. Nathan DM, Buse JB, Davidson MB, et al. Management of hyperglycemia in type 2 diabetes: a consensus algorithm for the initiation and adjustment of therapy: a consensus statement from the American Diabetes Association and the European Association for the Study of Diabetes. Diabetes Care 2006;29:1963–72.

Public Health Implications: Translation into Diabetes Prevention Initiatives—Four-Level Public Health Concept

Peter E.H. Schwarz, MD, PhD

KEYWORDS

- Diabetes prevention • Public health policy
- Implementation • Toolkit

The steady increase in the incidence of type 2 diabetes is a major challenge to health care systems and health policy development.[1] Diabetes leads to significantly reduced quality of life and life expectancy because of life-threatening comorbidities and complications.[2] Intriguingly, the disease is gaining strength and numbers in younger people,[3] resulting in an enormous impact on economic growth.

The most effective way to manage diabetes and its complications is to prevent its development in the first place. Recent studies have conclusively demonstrated that preventive approaches delay the onset of diabetes or prevent its development.[4–7] Intervention strategies addressing diet and exercise may reduce the relative risk of developing diabetes by 58% and pharmacologic treatment by 25% to 30%, with a more pronounced reduction in cardiovascular risk.[4,6,8] Economic evaluation has demonstrated the cost effectiveness of primary prevention of type 2 diabetes.[9] Despite the evidence, it remains questionable whether these programs are feasible at a population level.[10,11] The challenge, therefore, is to establish a scientifically based structural framework for efficiently managing nationwide prevention programs.[12,13]

DIABETES PREVENTION IN PRACTICE: A GLOBAL PANORAMA

In the last decade, several initiatives implemented evidence-based diabetes prevention programs based on large trials as well as experience from screening and behavior

Department for Prevention and Care of Diabetes, Medical Clinic III, University Clinic Carl Gustav Carus at the Technical University Dresden, Fetscherstraße 74, 01307 Dresden, Germany
E-mail address: peter.schwarz@uniklinikum-dresden.de

Med Clin N Am 95 (2011) 397–407
doi:10.1016/j.mcna.2010.11.008   medical.theclinics.com
0025-7125/11/$ – see front matter © 2011 Elsevier Inc. All rights reserved.

modification techniques. Thus, practice initiatives were developed on different formats and scales. Whereas some initiatives focused on established study designs and were implemented in a well-defined, structured setting, others expanded screening to reach large populations extrapolating from interventions in randomized controlled trials (RCTs). A recent publication describes screening and intervention procedures that were adapted to specific cultural settings with the goal of implementing programs on a national scale.[14] **Table 1** provides an overview of current large scale implementation trials and programs for diabetes prevention.

As the number of individuals who are at increased risk for developing diabetes involved in the referenced programs is still relatively small, it is very difficult to assess their impact. Using a scientific, outcome-driven perspective, most implementation trials failed, because they were unable to reach the same outcome as established trials or the outcome was not measured. From a health economics point of view, these initiatives were successful because they had a positive outcome and required considerably fewer resources than anticipated. From a public health perspective, these initiatives were highly effective, because they imparted knowledge of diabetes prevention and practice and identified barriers, difficulties, and challenges to implementation. Finally, aside from generating knowledge, the trial educated staff involved and provided valuable experience for planning prospective programs.

Experience from previous failures in implementation was especially helpful for improving future prevention initiatives. One such project, the European DE-PLAN (Diabetes in Europe-Prevention using Lifestyle, Physical Activity and Nutritional intervention) project,[15] consisted of 17 different prevention initiatives pursuing a common strategy. Several projects recently published their outcome data that achieved respectable results.[16] The major benefit of the DEPLAN project was the recognition of barriers for implementation related to challenging objectives and selecting proper indicators for the successful establishment of a practical diabetes prevention initiative in a public health setting.

EVIDENCE FOR PREVENTION PRACTICE

One of the major difficulties in translating knowledge generated by RCTs is the inability to generalize to the practice setting as they were conducted in a controlled environment. Greater resources were available for clinical trials than for practice programs, enabling the development of an ideal intervention structure. Attempting to translate interventions from studies into a practical setting with less funding led to deviations from the initial intervention protocols and generated a variety of new approaches.[17] These produced new intervention strategies and program milestones and confirmed the absolute necessity of developing practical guidelines for the implementation of diabetes prevention programs. This has currently been addressed in the IMAGE (Development and Implementation of a European Guideline and Training Standards for Diabetes Prevention) project.[15]

INTERVENTION MANAGER TRAINING

Another valuable lesson learned was the importance of intervention manager training. Most intervention managers had a background in diabetes education and applied this experience to prevention programs. In some settings, structured intervention programs and patient as well as trainer materials were developed. It seemed that the more intervention managers focused on behavioral and lifestyle changes (and less on diabetes education), the more successful they were. Furthermore, the availability of structured material was vital for an intervention to be successful. From these experiences, the European initiative, IMAGE, found it necessary to develop a curriculum for training prevention managers. The aim of this project was to disseminate knowledge and experience in intervention practice, to standardize educational requirements for prevention managers, and to emphasize strategies for behavioral change and motivation with less emphasis on diabetes education.[18]

QUALITY INDICATORS FOR DIABETES PREVENTION

A clear barrier for assessing diabetes prevention practice programs was the lack of adequate performance indicators. This deficiency was recognized early, but as a variety of indicators were implemented globally, standardization was lacking. Some groups attempted to evaluate program performance based on the oral glucose tolerance test (OGTT), similar to RCTs. Lack of funding and impracticality of performing the OGTT in a public health setting led to limited participation and unconvincing results. Other groups evaluated outcome based on behavioral change, weight loss, or reduction in waist circumference but were unable to stratify their results compared with RCTs. This inability demonstrates the dilemma of attempting to extrapolate results from RCTs into a public health care setting, which requires a completely different environment and different structures.

RCTs are characterized by scientific validity, with the primary objective of demonstrating adequate outcome of prespecified endpoints. In a public health setting, the primary goal, however, focuses on implementation of an intervention in a sizable population of eligible individuals. Therefore, scientific evaluation standards in RCTs need to be translated into the public health care setting with careful management of considerably more limited resources. Public health care interventions require outcome comparisons with RCTs by the use of defined indicators achieved by the international IMAGE consortium with a quality management structure.[19]

Quality indicators are targeted towards individuals responsible for diabetes prevention at 3 different levels of the health care system, namely the macro, meso, and micro levels. At the "macro" level, indicators apply to decision makers at the national level, generating the prerequisites for diabetes/obesity prevention. Examples of indicators at this level include prevalence of diabetes in the population and percentage of the population physically inactive. The "meso" level refers to the operative primary health care provider. Depending on the country, indicators may be used by individuals who are responsible for diabetes prevention in municipalities, health districts, health care centers, occupational health, the private sector, or at the local nongovernmental organizational level. Examples of indicators at the meso level include proportion of the population screened by health care providers per year and the percentage of identified high-risk individuals directed to diagnostic procedures. At the "micro" level, indicators are meant for personnel charged with executing the actual preventive work, which include physicians, nurses, dieticians, physiotherapists, or prevention managers. Examples of indicators at this level include change in waist circumference and quality of nutrition over 1 year.[19]

TARGET POPULATION

What is the appropriate target population for an intervention program for the primary prevention of type 2 diabetes? In the past, most RCTs studied subjects with impaired glucose tolerance diagnosed with independent tests. Translation of intervention strategies into a public health setting requires a clear definition of individuals at risk[20,21] and screening procedures that are efficient and easy to implement. This requirement poses a dilemma as eligibility criteria for intervention in RCTs were well defined,

Table 1
Public health diabetes prevention initiatives with potential on a national scale

Program	Aim	National Policy	Setting	Target Population	Intervention Manager	Intervention Program	Outcome Evaluation	Quality Management	Funding	References
FIND2D, Finland	Primary diabetes prevention	Yes – National Diabetes Plan	PHC, decentralized community	Person at risk FINDRISK >15	Diabetes nurses	1–3 sessions	Waist circ	None	National program	14,33
GOAL-LIT, Finland	Diabetes prevention and healthy ageing	Yes – National Diabetes Plan	PHC, decentralized, occupational medicine	Person at risk FINDRISK >12	Occupational nurses	5 sessions and 1 booster session	Anthr., biomarker, behavior by physician	None	Included in occupational service	34
PLAN4WARD, USA	Primary diabetes prevention	National Coordinating Center in Development	YMCA	American Diabetes Association Risk Score	Nonspecialist staff at YMCA	6-month, 16-session curriculum, then monthly maintenance sessions	Anthr., HbA1c, lipids	Centralized instructor training; peer-based session fidelity checklists	National Institutes of Health	11,35,36
Reset Your Life, Australia	People	Council of Australian Government	PHC, decentralized community	Person aged 40–49 years at risk AUSDRISK >12	Health professional	5 + 1 sessions, intervention facilitator	Waist and weight	None	Australian government	14
LIFE! Taking Action on Diabetes, Australia	Primary diabetes prevention	State Government of Victoria	PHC, decentralized community	Person at risk AUSDRISK >12	Health professional	5 + 1 sessions, intervention facilitator	Anthr., biomarker, behavior	Yes, at facilitator and program levels	Free for most participants aged 50 years or older	14
SDPP,[a] Australia	Primary diabetes prevention	NSW Department of Health	PHC, decentralized medical GP-based community	Person aged 50–65 years at risk AUSDRISK >15	Health professional	5 + 1 sessions, GP and lifestyle officer	Anthr., biomarker, behavior	None	NSW Department of Health	14
SDPP,[b] Germany	Primary diabetes prevention	Saxony, Gesundheitsziele	Public health, paramedical, decentralized community	Person at risk FINDRISK >10	Prevention manager, different professions	Structured program 8 sessions, telephone and email support and annual follow-up	Blood pressure, waist, anthr., parallel study on OGTT	Blood pressure and waist circ	Local health insurances reimburses prevention manager	10,14

Program	Aim	Local health policy	Setting	Risk factors evaluation	Health workers	Intervention	Outcome measures	Control group	Quality assurance	Funding	Ref
Do It Yourself, Canada	Diabetes prevention and management		Community, Aborigines		Health workers	3-day agenda + manual	None	None		Government + private	14
Walking Away from Type 2 Diabetes, UK	Primary diabetes prevention	National Health Service (NHS) Health Check Program	Primary care	High-risk person identified using the Leicester Risk Score	Registered or nonregistered health care professional	3.5-hour structured education program followed by annual maintenance program. Telephone contact every 6 months	1st = physical activity 2nd = OGTT, progression to diabetes, lipids and anthr. variables	None	All educators are trained and quality assured to ensure fidelity to Person-centered philosophy and content	Collaboration for Leadership in Applied Health Research and Care, National Institute for Health Research	37,38
Let's Prevent Diabetes, UK	Primary diabetes prevention	NHS Health Check Program	Primary care	Leicester Risk Score and confirmed with OGTT	Registered health care professional	6-hour structured education program followed by annual maintenance program. Telephone contact every 3 months	1st = progression to type 2 diabetes using OGTT 2nd = physical activity, diet, lipids, and anthr. variables	None	All educators are trained and quality assured to ensure fidelity to person-centered philosophy and content	National Institute for Health Research	14
Let's Beat Diabetes, New Zealand	Diabetes prevention and improved management of disease	National Strategy Healthy Eating Healthy Action (HEHA)	Community	Maori, Pacific, and South Asian with risk factors identification	At all levels from community people to health professionals	A range of different interventions are offered	Waist and weight	Yes	Yes	Regional funding from Health Budget and other partner organizations	14
DE-PLAN, Greece	Primary diabetes prevention		PHC, occupational	Person at risk FINDRISK >12	Prevention manager, nurse	6 sessions, by prevention manager	Blood pressure, waist, anthr., lipids, parallel study on OGTT	Parallel to intervention	Parallel to intervention	Public health + private	16

Abbreviations: Anthr., anthropomentric; AUSDRISK, The Australian Type 2 Diabetes Risk Assessment Tool; circ, circumference; GP, general practitioner; PHC, primary health care; YMCA, Young Men's Christian Association hostels.

[a] Sydney Diabetes Prevention Program.

[b] Saxony Diabetes Prevention Program.

allowing for time consuming and costly diagnostic procedures. From the public health perspective, however, it is mandatory to have valid, simple, and cost-effective screening or diagnostic tests that possess a high probability of identifying individuals at risk and can motivate them to participate in an intervention program. OGTT is the gold standard for diagnosing those at risk for diabetes; however, as it requires standardization and may not be cost effective, the OGTT may not be suitable for population screening.

Another approach for patient screening involves the use of risk scores.[20] Several scores have been developed, some only using anthropometric parameters (eg, waist circumference, body weight), which are ideal for self-assessment, whereas others used a combination of self-assessment– and laboratory-based parameters.[22–24] All of these scores provide a probability for predicting disease development.[25] However, public health–based evaluation of risk scores for screening demonstrated that although these tools may be feasible, they do not provide the necessary motivation for participation in an intervention program.

New diagnostic tools were developed in parallel that diagnose diabetes risk based on noninvasive techniques[26] or new risk management models based on HbA1c[27,28] and 1-hour postload glucose values.[29] Thus, there is no single ideal tool for assessing diabetes risk or identifying individuals with increased metabolic risk factors in a population-based public health setting. To conduct an intervention program, it is necessary to select among existing diagnostic or screening procedures appropriate for the setting based on cost and acceptability to the target population. These parameters define the target population and the number of eligible individuals suitable for intervention.

THE RELEVANCE OF NATIONAL POLICY INVOLVEMENT

Political support for establishing the framework for diabetes prevention programs is extremely important and mandatory for national implementation.[30] The driving force for a positive outcome includes the structure, transparency, daily life relevance of the intervention, and practicality of the program. The global experience of diabetes prevention programs demonstrated that a lack of political support or endorsement by stakeholders predicted little chance of achieving public health relevance. For successful national public health implementation, it is absolutely necessary to involve relevant stakeholders in the political arena, health insurance companies supporting nongovernmental organizations, the scientific community, and the target population. Within the European Union, only 5 of 27 countries have a national diabetes plan and only 1 has a national diabetes prevention program.[30] In Asia, the situation is similar, with a progressive increase in the number of countries including diabetes prevention in their national policies. The United States is at the forefront of governmental initiatives for developing a diabetes prevention program, with the Centers for Disease Control and Prevention being the driving force for coordinating the national effort. The existence of a national policy for supporting diabetes prevention does not equate with a positive outcome, but it is a mandatory first step for successful public health implementation.

FOUR-LEVEL PUBLIC HEALTH MODEL FOR IMPLEMENTATION OF DIABETES PREVENTION PROGRAMS

Diabetes prevention programs in clinical and public health practices have provided a variety of experiences over the past years, identifying different milestones and roadblocks that are essential for ensuring successful program implementation (**Fig. 1**).[30] Also, there are different levels in the public health environment required for

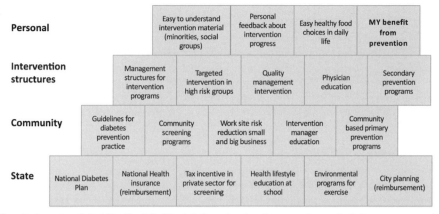

Fig. 1. Four-level Public Health Model for the implementation of diabetes prevention programs.

implementing a national program including state and governmental sectors necessary to create awareness and a suitable political environment. The community level, responsible for implementation, requires educational components and guidelines for screening. Structures, the next level, are important for the development of diabetes prevention programs achievable only in the context of a comprehensive prevention organization. They are also necessary to assure quality program management, to involve physician education, as well as to establish a link to secondary prevention programs. The last level in this model is the personal level that addresses the need, attitude, and behavior of those considered at increased risk (see **Fig. 1**).

State Level

The state level, represented by governmental stakeholders, is critical for policy development. A national diabetes plan including a prevention strategy establishes the public health framework for implementation. As a part of this plan, national or local health insurances should be involved and adequate reimbursement needs to be assured. A structured plan for screening and instructing healthy behavior, exercise, and physical activity is required. Furthermore, healthy lifestyle education introduced in schools, especially in primary schools, would build the basis for sustainability over a life time and decrease the burden of obesity and type 2 diabetes. The state level is, therefore, the basis for primary diabetes prevention public health activities, and it assures the effectiveness of an intervention program.

Community Level

The community has the highest responsibility for implementing an intervention program and provides the underlying structural platform. The community builds the framework for network structures, screening and intervention programs, "and" raus providing healthy food choices Komma raus and supporting physical activity. Establishing a healthy work place environment is difficult, especially for small businesses, but this would be of value for public health by reducing risk for metabolic diseases at the work site.

Intervention Structures

Intervention depends on a program management structure; evidence-based practice has its strongest impact at this level. If the community is able to establish the corridor through which the intervention can be performed, the relevant structures must be established. Success of the program will depend on intervention management as well as the degree of networking in the community. There must be clear guidance for prevention practice and intervention program development for targeting high-risk groups. Quality management in the intervention process requires routine reporting of program performance and accomplishments to stakeholders at the state level and is mandatory to secure further support. Furthermore, quality management can be used as an indicator for assessing performance. If the intervention is organized in a medical setting, physician involvement, relevant physician education, as well as networking with available secondary prevention programs are necessary.

Personal Level

The personal level is critical as it pertains to those at increased risk and therefore eligible for intervention. This level is the overall indicator of the program's quality and success if all other levels have been adequately addressed. The individual will be motivated to participate if the benefit of the prevention program is easily comprehensible and if barriers for participation are eliminated. This applies especially to minorities or ethnic groups in the community setting. Easily comprehensible intervention materials are critical to foster participation with solicitation of feedback to further improve adherence to the program and lifestyle change. The personal level will be benefited as well by any activity that makes it easier to adopt healthy food choices.

The four-level public health model requires milestones to develop an effective prevention program. Failing to address 1 milestone can result in roadblocks for program management and implementation. Milestones are generally not stand-alone milestones and are highly interrelated. This makes the initial effort challenging, but progression from one milestone or level to the next becomes easier as incremental progress is achieved. This public health model is applicable to most westernized health care systems and can be adapted to others. The most important issue to address relates to the personal benefits that eligible individuals derive from the intervention. If this is made comprehensible on an individual level and achievable in the short-term level, the likelihood for successful implementation of a diabetes prevention program is high.

PRACTICAL GUIDANCE FOR PREVENTION OF DIABETES

The IMAGE Study Group systematically assembled information from clinical trials as well as from "real world" implementation programs. Approximately 100 European experts worked for more than 2 years to prepare the main deliverables of the project, which include evidence-based guidelines for type 2 diabetes prevention,[31] a toolkit,[32] a guideline for evaluation, as well as quality indicators and management for type 2 diabetes prevention.[19] Furthermore, a European training curriculum was developed for prevention managers. The next step requires development of national action plans for diabetes prevention involving stakeholders at governmental and nongovernmental levels as well as scientific and practical guidance. The action plan needs to identify essential activities and available resources for diabetes prevention and elucidate the responsibilities of each stakeholder. In addition, the plan needs to recommend and outline action steps specific to each cohort involved (eg, families, friends, health care providers, the media, health insurance providers, employers, researchers, professional educators, ethnic and cultural groups and so on).

TOOLKIT FOR THE PREVENTION OF TYPE 2 DIABETES

The major output of the IMAGE project relevant for prevention practice is the practical guideline called "Toolkit for the prevention of type 2 diabetes." The toolkit is meant for all involved with diabetes prevention: not only those working in primary and specialized health care services, physicians, physical activity experts, dieticians, nurses, and teachers but also stakeholders and politicians. The IMAGE toolkit provides practical information for preventive intervention for adults at risk for developing diabetes. The toolkit includes in a condensed form the essence of what is necessary to develop a diabetes prevention program covering management, financial, intervention, and quality assurance aspects and refers to the latest evidence from the science of diabetes prevention and translates this knowledge into practice. The toolkit also contains practical examples and worksheets that facilitate implementation.

The toolkit addresses issues such as budgeting, financing, and identifying individuals at risk. The core of the toolkit describes elements of an effective lifestyle intervention program. A process for supporting lifestyle behavior change is described in its phases (motivation, action, and maintenance). It describes the core goals of lifestyle modification (physical activity and diet) and gives practical instruction for addressing these with the client. Other behaviors considered in diabetes prevention include smoking, stress or depression, and sleeping patterns. The toolkit provides an overview on evaluating intervention programs, establishing quality assurance, and several recommendations that help with planning type 2 diabetes prevention programs. The International Diabetes Federation estimates that the number of patients with type 2 diabetes is likely to increase in forthcoming years and perhaps decades in Europe. However, with implementing recommendations from the IMAGE project, the prevention of type 2 diabetes can become a reality, and the diabetes epidemic may eventually be controlled and its burden gradually diminished.

NETWORK: "WHO ARE ACTIVE IN DIABETES PREVENTION"

An important current initiative is the implementation of an international network "Who are active in diabetes prevention" for those who wish to become involved in the prevention of diabetes and facilitates networking with others sharing a common interest. The network, although encouraging the exchange of knowledge, recent intervention material, as well as educational standards, focuses most on the exchange of experiences from diabetes prevention practices. It is also a vehicle for exchanging scientific information among research groups, those interested in diabetes prevention or active in practice. An international exchange of ideas regarding diabetes prevention practice will help develop improved prevention programs and reduce barriers and mistakes. Participants from more than 135 countries are already part of the network, especially many from low- and middle-income countries. Individuals interested are invited to register without charge and to benifit from this global network at www.activeindiabetesprevention.com.

REFERENCES

1. Zimmet P, Alberti KG, Shaw J. Global and societal implications of the diabetes epidemic. Nature 2001;414(6865):782–7.
2. Zimmet P, Shaw J, Alberti KG. Preventing type 2 diabetes and the dysmetabolic syndrome in the real world: a realistic view. Diabet Med 2003;20(9):693–702.
3. Nestle M. Preventing childhood diabetes: the need for public health intervention. Am J Public Health 2005;95(9):1497–9.
4. Knowler WC, Barrett-Connor E, Fowler SE, et al. Reduction in the incidence of type 2 diabetes with lifestyle intervention or metformin. N Engl J Med 2002; 346(6):393–403.

5. Tuomilehto J, Lindström J, Eriksson JG, et al. Prevention of type 2 diabetes mellitus by changes in lifestyle among subjects with impaired glucose tolerance. N Engl J Med 2001;344(18):1343–50.

6. Chiasson JL, Josse RG, Gomis R, et al. Acarbose for prevention of type 2 diabetes mellitus: the STOP-NIDDM randomised trial. Lancet 2002;359(9323):2072–7.

7. Pan XR, Li GW, Hu YH, et al. Effects of diet and exercise in preventing NIDDM in people with impaired glucose tolerance. The Da Qing IGT and Diabetes Study. Diabetes Care 1997;20(4):537–44.

8. Torgerson JS, Hauptman J, Boldrin MN, et al. XENical in the prevention of diabetes in obese subjects (XENDOS) study: a randomized study of orlistat as an adjunct to lifestyle changes for the prevention of type 2 diabetes in obese patients. Diabetes Care 2004;27(1):155–61.

9. Hernan WH, Brandle M, Zhang P, et al. Costs associated with the primary prevention of type 2 diabetes mellitus in the diabetes prevention program. Diabetes Care 2003;26(1):36–47.

10. Schwarz PE, Schwarz J, Schuppenies A, et al. Development of a diabetes prevention management program for clinical practice. Public Health Rep 2007; 122(2):258–63.

11. Ackermann RT, Marrero DG. Adapting the Diabetes Prevention Program lifestyle intervention for delivery in the community: the YMCA model. Diabetes Educ 2007; 33(1):69, 74–5, 77–8.

12. Tuomilehto J, Schwarz PE. Primary prevention of type 2 diabetes is advancing towards the mature stage in Europe. Horm Metab Res 2010;42(Suppl 1):1–2.

13. Rothe U, Müller G, Schwarz PE, et al. Evaluation of a diabetes management system based on practice guidelines, integrated care, and continuous quality management in a Federal State of Germany: a population-based approach to health care research. Diabetes Care 2008;31(5):863–8.

14. Schwarz PE, Greaves C, Reddy P, et al. Diabetes prevention in practice, vol. 1. Dresden (Germany): TUMAINI Institute for Prevention management; 2010. p. 232.

15. Schwarz PE, Lindström J, Kissimova-Scarbeck K, et al. The European perspective of type 2 diabetes prevention: diabetes in Europe–prevention using lifestyle, physical activity and nutritional intervention (DE-PLAN) project. Exp Clin Endocrinol Diabetes 2008;116(3):167–72.

16. Makrilakis K, Liatis S, Grammatikou S, et al. Implementation and effectiveness of the first community lifestyle intervention programme to prevent type 2 diabetes in Greece. The DE-PLAN study. Diabet Med 2010;27(4):459–65.

17. O'Gorman DJ, Krook A. Exercise and the treatment of diabetes and obesity. Endocrinol Metab Clin North Am 2008;37(4):887–903.

18. Schwarz PE, Gruhl U, Bornstein SR, et al. The European Perspective on Diabetes Prevention: development and Implementation of a European Guideline and training standards for diabetes prevention (IMAGE). Diab Vasc Dis Res 2007; 4(4):353–7.

19. Pajunen P, Landgraf R, Muylle F, et al. Quality indicators for the prevention of type 2 diabetes in Europe–IMAGE. Horm Metab Res 2010;42(Suppl 1):S56–63.

20. Schwarz PE, Li J, Lindstrom J, et al. Tools for predicting the risk of type 2 diabetes in daily practice. Horm Metab Res 2009;41(2):86–97.

21. Inzucchi SE, Sherwin RS. The prevention of type 2 diabetes mellitus. Endocrinol Metab Clin North Am 2005;34(1):199–219, viii.

22. Al-Lawati JA, Tuomilehto J. Diabetes risk score in Oman: a tool to identify prevalent type 2 diabetes among Arabs of the Middle East. Diabetes Res Clin Pract 2007;77(3):438–44.

23. Rathmann W, Martin S, Haastert B, et al. Performance of screening question-naires and risk scores for undiagnosed diabetes: the KORA Survey 2000. Arch Intern Med 2005;165(4):436–41.
24. Schwarz PE, Li J, Reimann M, et al. The finnish diabetes risk score is associated with insulin resistance and progression towards type 2 diabetes. J Clin Endocri-nol Metab 2009;94(3):920–6.
25. Glumer C, Vistisen D, Borch-Johnsen K, et al. Risk scores for type 2 diabetes can be applied in some populations but not all. Diabetes Care 2006;29(2):410–4.
26. Ramachandran A, Moses A, Shetty S, et al. A new non-invasive technology to screen for dysglycaemia including diabetes. Diabetes Res Clin Pract 2010;88: 302–6.
27. Ziemer DC, Kolm P, Weintraub WS, et al. Glucose-independent, black-white differences in hemoglobin A1c levels: a cross-sectional analysis of 2 studies. Ann Intern Med 2010;152(12):770–7.
28. Bergman M. Inadequacies of absolute threshold levels for diagnosing predia-betes. Diabetes Metab Res Rev 2010;26(1):3–6.
29. Abdul-Ghani MA, Lyssenko V, Tuomi T, et al. Fasting versus postload plasma glucose concentration and the risk for future type 2 diabetes: results from the Bot-nia Study. Diabetes Care 2009;32(2):281–6.
30. Schwarz PE, Muylle F, Valensi P, et al. The European perspective of diabetes prevention. Horm Metab Res 2008;40(8):511–4.
31. Paulweber B, Valensi P, Lindström J, et al. A European evidence-based guideline for the prevention of type 2 diabetes. Horm Metab Res 2010;42(Suppl 1):S3–36.
32. Lindstrom J, Neumann A, Sheppard KE, et al. Take action to prevent diabetes–the IMAGE toolkit for the prevention of type 2 diabetes in Europe. Horm Metab Res 2010;42(Suppl 1):S37–55.
33. Saaristo T, Peltonen M, Keinänen-Kiukaanniemi S, et al. National type 2 diabetes prevention programme in Finland: FIN-D2D. Int J Circumpolar Health 2007;66(2): 101–12.
34. Absetz P, Valve R, Oldenburg B, et al. Type 2 diabetes prevention in the "real world": one-year results of the GOAL implementation trial. Diabetes Care 2007; 30(10):2465–70.
35. Ackermann RT, Finch EA, Brizendine E, et al. Translating the Diabetes Prevention Program into the community. The DEPLOY Pilot Study. Am J Prev Med 2008; 35(4):357–63.
36. Lipscomb ER, Finch EA, Brizendine E, et al. Reduced 10-year risk of coronary heart disease in patients who participated in a community-based diabetes prevention program: the DEPLOY pilot study. Diabetes Care 2009;32(3):394–6.
37. Yates T, Davies M, Gorely T, et al. Effectiveness of a pragmatic education program designed to promote walking activity in individuals with impaired glucose tolerance: a randomized controlled trial. Diabetes Care 2009;32(8): 1404–10.
38. Yates T, Davies M, Gorely T, et al. Rationale, design and baseline data from the Pre-diabetes Risk Education and Physical Activity Recommendation and Encour-agement (PREPARE) programme study: a randomized controlled trial. Patient Educ Couns 2008;73(2):264–71.

Glycemic Status, Metabolic Syndrome, and Cardiovascular Risk in Children

Gerald S. Berenson, MD[a],*, Mehmet Agirbasli, MD[b],
Quoc Manh Nguyen, MD, MPH[a], Wei Chen, MD, PhD[a],
Sathanur R. Srinivasan, PhD[a]

KEYWORDS

• Obesity • Diabetes • Cardiovascular • Risk factor

Carbohydrate-insulin imbalance underlying atherosclerosis, hypertension, and diabetes mellitus has become one of the most common causes of death in the United States.[1,2] The epidemic of childhood obesity is contributing to this population problem, and if proper precautions are not taken, obesity, and often associated diabetes, has the potential to reverse the gains made in the twentieth century in cardiovascular (CV) disease prevention.[3,4] Alarming increases in obesity might even impact cancer incidence. Obesity turns out to be the major causal factor for this carbohydrate-insulin imbalance and the clinical states designated as prediabetes and diabetes mellitus in the US population.[5] Therefore, understanding the underlying risk factors for the disturbed entity of cardiometabolic syndrome and strategies to address contributing risk factors are desperately needed. To develop a comprehensive approach to the prevention of this problem should be a high priority of the medical community.

With regard to the progressive global epidemic of obesity, the worldwide prevalence of type 2 diabetes will increase by 50% to 360 million over the next 30 years.[6] This global problem will cause an even much larger population to be classified as prediabetic. Additional risk of CV mortality outcomes is destined to occur. The natural history of the cardiometabolic syndrome and its relationship with diabetic status is increasingly

This study was supported by grants AG-16592 from the National Institute on Aging, HD-061437 and HD-062783 from the National Institute of Child Health and Human Development, 0855082E from the American Heart Association, and 546145G1 from the Tulane University.
Conflict of interest: The authors have no conflict of interest.
[a] Tulane Center for Cardiovascular Health, Tulane University Health Sciences Center, 1440 Canal Street, Suite 1829, New Orleans, LA 70112, USA
[b] Department of Cardiology, Marmara University, Istanbul, Turkey
* Corresponding author.
E-mail address: berenson@tulane.edu

Med Clin N Am 95 (2011) 409–417
doi:10.1016/j.mcna.2010.11.011
0025-7125/11/$ – see front matter © 2011 Published by Elsevier Inc.

understood. From long-term studies beginning in childhood, it is now clear that these abnormal metabolic and physiologic characteristics are evident in early life.[7,8]

EPIDEMIOLOGIC TRENDS OF OBESITY AND ITS MEASUREMENT

An adverse outcome of unhealthy lifestyles in our population and in early life is the onset of obesity. Obesity (this term is used generically for adiposity to include over-weight and obesity according to the Centers for Disease Control and Prevention [CDC] standards) is now so common in our population and worldwide and is attracting broad public health attention. Obesity is related to both a genetic predisposition and a balance between energy intake and energy expenditure and an interaction with environmentally determined life styles. The secular trend of obesity in our society has occurred in populations, with the same genetic pool implicating environmental factors that determine this trend.

Although approximately 40% of our population has become obese by adolescence and young adulthood, the trend of increasing obesity has continued.[9] To illustrate changes occurring in South America, a recent study of children and adolescents in the age group of 10 to 15 years in Brazil indicates an increase in the body mass index (BMI, calculated as the weight in kilograms divided by the height in meters squared) of 2.5 units in girls and 5.0 units in boys.[10] This increase was observed in a multiracial population that demonstrates a propensity to develop obesity despite ethnic differences. In the Bogalusa Heart Study of a biracial (black/white) population representing the southeastern United States, white boys showed a greater increase in obesity rate, especially in adolescence and young adulthood, whereas black girls showed the greatest overall increase. Obesity in black girls begins at puberty around 8 years of age and notoriously accelerates into adulthood.[11]

Childhood obesity interacts with other CV risk factors and becomes a prime determinant of hypertension, dyslipidemia, and diabetes mellitus. Obesity in childhood is the most consistent predictor of adult heart disease.[12] CV risk becomes abnormal around the 85th percentile of body weight, a level well below the 95th percentile that is considered alarming by the CDC.[13] At this level, lower high-density lipoprotein cholesterol (HDL-C), higher triglycerides, and other risk factor changes along with CV system changes are observed by noninvasive methods.

INTERRELATION OF CV RISK FACTORS

Risk factors tend to cluster and aggregate and have an interactive and additive affect on CV risk. As described in Framingham, MA, an increase in the number of risk factors is associated with increased CV events and mortality. Observations in the Bogalusa Heart Study have elaborated race/gender differences in children and adolescents in the aggregation of risk factors.[14] For example, white children, having greater fat mass in early life, show a stronger relation to higher blood pressure levels, faster heart rates, and higher glucose levels.[15,16] Considerable changes occur during puberty with a decrease in HDL-C levels and an increase in low-density lipoprotein cholesterol levels in adolescence and young adulthood in white boys.[14] These changes in lipoprotein levels may account for the greater coronary atherosclerosis observed in white boys associated with earlier coronary events in contrast to black boys.

IMPLICATION OF ABNORMAL RISK FACTORS

The most dramatic example of the effects of risk factor clustering is from autopsy studies indicating that the confluence of several factors lead to the involvement and acceleration of atherosclerotic lesions in the coronary arteries.[17] Fibrous plaque lesions, which can progress, show significant correlation with multiple risk factors. There are methods that, at present, can be applied that measure silent changes within the CV system. The frequently used echo Doppler method applies ultrasonic measurement of the heart and blood vessels, especially carotid artery assessment for carotid intima-media thickness (IMT), as a surrogate of coronary artery disease. The bulb or bifurcation region relates more to multiple risk factors. **Fig. 1** illustrates that carotid IMT demonstrating greater degree of atherosclerosis is associated with a greater number of risk factors.[18] The percentile IMT change related to age can be used as a vascular score, which can complement the Framingham chronologic age score.[19]

There are other instruments that provide data on changes occurring in the CV system. Compliance or distensibility of brachial arteries while recording blood pressure is of particular use and similar measures can be used to study endothelial function.[20–22] Other instruments can provide measures related to vascular stiffness, such as pulse wave velocity, reflecting the effects of hypertensive atherosclerotic

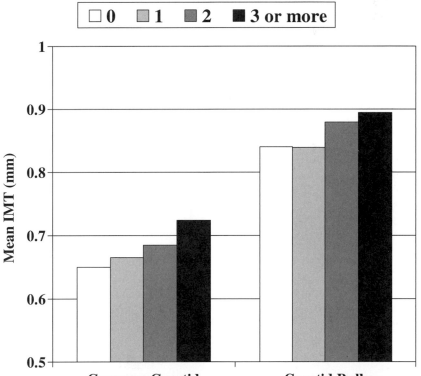

Fig. 1. Increasing carotid IMT related to increasing number of risk factors. The effect of multiple risk factors on the IMT of carotid artery segments in young adults. A highly significant trend of increasing thickness is shown with greater numbers of risk factors. Risk factors included were total cholesterol to HDL-C ratio, waist circumference, systolic blood pressure, insulin level (>75th percentile specific for age, race, and gender), and smoking. (*From* Urbina EM, Srinivasan SR, Tang R, et al. Impact of multiple coronary risk factors on the intima-media thickness of different segments of carotid artery in healthy young adults (The Bogalusa Heart Study). Am J Cardiol 2002;90:958; with permission.)

disease.[23] These measures provide clues to the damage and burden from risk factors. Because these measures can be obtained in young individuals, they provide evidence of risk factor burden over time.

The term deadly quartet aptly fits the classic 4 components of the syndrome X or metabolic syndrome as proposed by Reaven[24] in 1988.[25] Of these 4 components, central deposition of body fat, hyperinsulinemia, hypertension, and hypertriglyceridemia, the syndrome has been markedly expanded by largely understanding the role of each component, especially central body fat. The driving forces of the syndrome are obesity and hyperinsulinemia, which link hypertension with dyslipidemia. Studies have shown that childhood obesity precedes hyperinsulinemia before it manifests later in young adulthood.[26] Further, because BMI appreciably changes with growth of children, abdominal circumference related to increasing height (waist/height) is a good measure of central obesity.[27] Waist is to height ratio averages 0.5 at different ages and is a good reference complementing BMI.

METABOLIC SYNDROME IN CHILDREN

Although the metabolic syndrome was originally described in adults and is highly prevalent in older individuals, the coexistence of multiple CV risk factors also occurs commonly in children.[28,29] Multiple risk factors reinforce each other and persist (track) from childhood into adulthood. Studies suggest that the metabolic syndrome may even originate in the fetus.[30] In children with a BMI greater than 95 percentile, prevalence of the metabolic syndrome is 17.3% and clustering is strongly associated with insulin resistance measured by homeostasis model assessment.[31]

There remains some controversy regarding the definition of metabolic syndrome in adults. Several definitions have been proposed perhaps based on the differences of metabolic syndrome components in various ethnic groups. Several organizations, including the World Health Organization, the National Cholesterol Education Program, and the International Diabetes Foundation, have proposed different definitions of the metabolic syndrome in adults. Variable definitions account for differences in available data on its prevalence in various populations. There are no consistent criteria for diagnosing this condition in the pediatric age group. This diagnosis is further complicated by the changing levels of CV risk factors with growth and maturation. The prevalence of the metabolic syndrome phenotype in adolescents using the Bogalusa Heart Study data at different ages approximated 11% in the late 1990s.[32] Yet obesity, as pointed out, has continued to increase over the past 2 decades.[9] The authors propose a simple approach using the 75th percentile for its various components and the 25th percentile for HDL-C as shown in **Box 1**. These approximations for establishing the diagnosis in childhood gives greater credibility to prevalence estimates of diabetes and the metabolic syndrome in adults.[33]

Box 1
Criteria for metabolic syndrome in children

- Risk factors* greater than 75th percentiles (<25th percentile for HDL-C)

- Positive family history

- Obesity, dyslipidemia, hypertension, hyperinsulinemia. Select 3 or more risk factors but include at least 1 measure of obesity (eg, BMI, waist/height, circumference)

* Available population data: National Health and Nutrition Examination Survey,[34] Bogalusa Heart Study,[14] Muscatiine study,[35] Finnish Youth.[36]

Is the controversy on a precise definition worthwhile? Much has been learned about each of the original 4 components since the syndrome was proposed. Various names, such as cardiometabolic syndrome or insulin resistance syndrome, have been suggested. The involvement of the CV-renal systems is better understood as that of inflammatory components, which have added to the complexity of the syndrome (**Box 2**). Increased appreciation of lipotoxicity associated with fat accumulation in various organs and adipocyte generation of metabolic, hormonal, and inflammatory mediators has greatly expanded the significance of the syndrome.[37]

LONG-TERM CONSEQUENCES OF METABOLIC SYNDROME BEGINNING IN CHILDHOOD

In studies of children, it is important, particularly from the standpoint of prevention, to early evaluate the level of obesity by BMI and waist/height parameters as well as the carbohydrate-insulin metabolism status. The authors found parental history to contribute to findings of abnormal risk factors in offspring, especially diabetes mellitus.[38] In addition, the authors found fasting blood sugar level above the 50th percentile of 86 mg/dL to be a marker for the future development of prediabetes or

---

Box 2
Impact of obesity and related clinical CV-renal risk

Fat cell generated

    Inflammatory mediators

        Cytokines, TNF-α, IL-6 (CRP)

    Angiogenic proteins

        VEGF

    Metabolic regulators

        Adiponection

        Leptin

    Free fatty acids

    Angiotensinogen

    Stem cells

Obesity interrelationships

    Serum lipids and lipoproteins

    Hyperglycemia

    Hyperinsulinemia

    Diabetes

    Cardiovascular

        LVM, Cardiac dilatation

        Vascular stiffness

    Renal

        End stage renal disease

    Non-alcoholic fatty hepatitis

Abbreviations: CRP, C-reactive protein; LVM, left ventricular mass; TNF-α, tumor necrosis factor α; VEGF, vascular endothelial growth factor.

diabetes.[39] Childhood levels of glucose homeostasis in the top decile, homeostasis model assessment of insulin resistance, and insulin and glucose were 5.84, 5.54, and 3.28 times, respectively, and were particularly at risk for progression.[40] Children in the top decile were more likely to develop diabetes, and changes in the risk variables of the metabolic syndrome, including BMI, mean arterial blood pressure, HDL-C level, and triglyceride levels, predicted the onset of prediabetes and diabetes.[41]

INTERRELATION OF METABOLIC SYNDROME AND DIABETES STATUS

A common definition of metabolic syndrome in children remains unclear. Prediabetes and type 2 diabetes represent 2 categories of impaired glucose regulation and are associated with a constellation of disorders characteristic of the metabolic syndrome beginning in early life.[42,43] Consequently, it is obviously important to develop a consensus for the cutoff value of childhood fasting plasma glucose (FPG) level for predicting prediabetes and type 2 diabetes in adults. The FPG level has been proven to have high reproducibility, small variability, and favorable application to clinical settings.[44] After an average of 21 years of follow-up, in a multivariate analysis of repeated measurements adjusted for traditional risk factors, previous studies demonstrated that childhood FPG levels along with obesity, rather than fasting insulin levels, are the most important predictors of adult prediabetes and type 2 diabetes.[39]

Earlier novel proposals have questioned the adequacies of absolute threshold levels for diagnosing prediabetes. The current cutoff value for FPG (100 mg/dL) recommended by the American Diabetes Associations (ADA) is applied without distinction to age groups, even in the youth.[45] Moreover, the ADA asserts that risk for diabetes related to FPG is continuous. However, the authors' findings have suggested a threshold of 86 mg/dL in children above which the risk of adult diabetes begins to increase.[39] This finding is in agreement with an accompanying editorial by Gillman.[46]

The question of lowering the cutoff point for impaired FPG diagnosis in children to predict diabetes later in life is an interesting challenge that needs more long-term data beginning in childhood and is important in view of the public health crisis of obesity accompanied by underlying silent changes in the CV system.

IMPLICATION FOR PREVENTION

Observations in childhood suggest that the ability to predict prediabetes and diabetes is critical for their prevention early in life as well as for the prevention of CV diseases. The authors have been advocating the importance of prevention beginning in childhood particularly based on findings at autopsy. The authors propose introducing a comprehensive health promotion and education program beginning in kindergarten.[47] This program addresses the entire school environment, classroom, cafeteria, physical education, and role models (parents and teachers), and involves businesses, medical, and educational aspects of the community. The program the authors use is broad and emphasizes prevention not only of obesity but also of tobacco and alcohol use and social problems, such as violent behavior and dropouts. This program has been introduced in an entire Parish (County) to approximately 5000 school children as a model for other geographic areas.[48] In a school recording BMI and using the President's Fitness Challenge, data provided showed that weight reduction and improved quarter-mile run times were benefits of increased physical activity and education on nutrition. Many activities are included in the teaching process. By starting with school children, these activities become a public health approach to improving the health of individuals living in a toxic environment at a time when CV disease begins.

COMMENTS

The metabolic syndrome and adult manifestation of prediabetes and diabetes are major public health problems that begin in childhood. Prevention must be considered as a serious public health issue. Health education and health promotion of school children needs incorporation as a community effort.

ACKNOWLEDGMENTS

The authors wish to express their appreciation to the subjects in Bogalusa who have participated over a long period of time and for whom this study could not have been conducted without their support.

REFERENCES

1. Mokdad AH, Serdula MK, Dietz WH, et al. The continuing epidemic of obesity in the United States. JAMA 2000;284:1650–1.
2. Hoyert DL, Heron MP, Murphy SL, et al. Deaths. Final data for 2003. National vital statistics reports; vol. 54, No 13. Hyattsville (MD): National Center for Health Statistics; 2006.
3. Fox CS, Sullivan L, D'Agostino RB Sr, et al, Framingham Heart Study. The significant effect of diabetes duration on coronary heart disease mortality: the Framingham Heart Study. Diabetes Care 2004;27:704–8.
4. Olshansky SJ, Passaro DJ, Hershow RC, et al. A potential decline in life expectancy in the United States in the 21st century. N Engl J Med 2005;352:1138–45.
5. Cowie CC, Rust KF, Ford ES, et al. Full accounting of diabetes and pre-diabetes in the U.S. population in 1988–1994 and 2005–2006. Diabetes Care 2009;32: 287–94.
6. Wild S, Roglic G, Green A, et al. Global prevalence of diabetes: estimates for the year 2000 and projections for 2030. Diabetes Care 2004;27:1047–53.
7. Chen W, Berenson GS. Metabolic syndrome: definition and prevalence in children. J Pediatr (Rio J) 2007;83:1–2.
8. Agirbasli M, Agaoglu NB, Orak N, et al. Sex hormones, insulin resistance and high-density lipoprotein cholesterol levels in children. Horm Res Paediatr 2010; 73:166–74.
9. Broyles S, Katzmarzyk PT, Srinivasan SR, et al. The pediatric obesity epidemic continues unabated in Bogalusa, Louisiana. Pediatrics 2010;125:900–5.
10. Zanetti MA, Padua I, Branco LM, et al. Body mass index percentiles in adolescents of the city of Sao Paulo, Brazil, and their comparison with international parameters. Arq Bras Endocrinol Metabol 2010;54:295–302.
11. Webber LS, Cresanta JL, Croft JB, et al. Transitions of cardiovascular risk from adolescence to young adulthood—the Bogalusa Heart Study: II. Alterations in anthropometric blood pressure and serum lipoprotein variables. J Chronic Dis 1986;39:91–103.
12. Haji SA, Ulusoy RE, Patel DA, et al. Predictors of left ventricular dilatation in young adults (from the Bogalusa Heart Study). Am J Cardiol 2006;98:1234–7.
13. Freedman DS, Dietz WH, Srinivasan SR, et al. The relation of overweight to cardiovascular risk factors among children and adolescents: the Bogalusa Heart Study. Pediatrics 1999;103:1175–82.
14. Berenson GS. Causation of cardiovascular risk factors in children: perspective on cardiovascular risk in early life. New York: Raven Press; 1986.

15. Voors AW, Berenson GS, Dalferes ER, et al. Racial differences in blood pressure control. Science 1979;204:1091–4.
16. Berenson GS, Voors AW, Webber LS, et al. Racial differences of parameters associated with blood pressure levels in children—the Bogalusa Heart Study. Metabolism 1979;28:1218–28.
17. Berenson GS, Wattigney WA, Tracy RE, et al. Atherosclerosis of the aorta and coronary arteries and cardiovascular risk factors in persons aged 6 to 30 years and studied at necropsy (The Bogalusa Heart Study). Am J Cardiol 1992;70: 851–8.
18. Urbina EM, Srinivasan SR, Tang R, et al, Bogalusa Heart Study. Impact of multiple coronary risk factors on the intima-media thickness of different segments of carotid artery in healthy young adults (The Bogalusa Heart Study). Am J Cardiol 2002;90:953–8.
19. Tzou WS, Douglas PS, Srinivasan SR, et al. Distribution and predictors of carotid intima-media thickness in young adults. Prev Cardiol 2007;10:181–9.
20. Juonala M, Järvisalo MJ, Mäki-Torkko N, et al. Risk factors identified in childhood and decreased carotid artery elasticity in adulthood: the Cardiovascular Risk in Young Finns Study. Circulation 2005;112:1486–93.
21. Freedman DS, Patel DA, Srinivasan SR, et al. The contribution of childhood obesity to adult carotid intima-media thickness: the Bogalusa Heart Study. Int J Obes (Lond) 2008;32:749–56.
22. Urbina EM, Kimball TR, McCoy CE, et al. Youth with obesity and obesity-related type 2 diabetes mellitus demonstrate abnormalities in carotid structure and function. Circulation 2009;119:2913–9.
23. Li S, Chen W, Srinivasan SR, et al. Influence of metabolic syndrome on arterial stiffness and its age-related change in young adults: the Bogalusa Heart Study. Atherosclerosis 2005;180:349–54.
24. Reaven GM. Banting lecture 1988. Role of insulin resistance in human disease [review]. Diabetes 1988;37:1595–607.
25. Kaplan NM. The deadly quartet and the insulin resistance syndrome: an historical overview [review]. Hypertens Res 1996;19(Suppl 1):S9–11.
26. Srinivasan SR, Myers L, Berenson GS. Temporal association between obesity and hyperinsulinemia in children, adolescents, and young adults: the Bogalusa Heart Study. Metabolism 1999;48:928–34.
27. Srinivasan SR, Wang R, Chen W, et al. Utility of waist-to-height ratio in detecting central obesity and related adverse cardiovascular risk profile among normal weight younger adults (from the Bogalusa Heart Study). Am J Cardiol 2009;104:721–4.
28. Chen W, Srinivasan SR, Elkasabany A, et al. The association of cardiovascular risk factor clustering related to insulin resistance syndrome (Syndrome X) between young parents and their offspring: the Bogalusa Heart Study. Atherosclerosis 1999;145:197–205.
29. Pischon T, Boeing H, Hoffmann K, et al. General and abdominal adiposity and risk of death in Europe. N Engl J Med 2008;359:2105–20.
30. Barker DJ, Hales CN, Fall CH, et al. Type 2 (non-insulin-dependent) diabetes mellitus, hypertension and hyperlipidaemia (syndrome X): relation to reduced fetal growth. Diabetologia 1993;36:62–7.
31. Chen W, Srinivasan SR, Li S, et al. Clustering of long-term trends in metabolic syndrome variables from childhood to adulthood in Blacks and Whites: the Bogalusa Heart Study. Am J Epidemiol 2007;166(5):527–33.
32. Chen W, Bao W, Begum S, et al. Age-related patterns of the clustering of cardiovascular risk variables of syndrome X from childhood to young adulthood in

a population made up of black and white subjects: the Bogalusa Heart Study. Diabetes 2000;49:1042–8.

33. Molnár D. The prevalence of the metabolic syndrome and type 2 diabetes mellitus in children and adolescents. Int J Obes Relat Metab Disord 2004;28(Suppl 3): S70–4.

34. Available at: http://www.cdc.gov/nchs/nhanes/bibliograph/default.aspx. Accessed November 12, 2010.

35. Lauer RM, Burns T, Daniels SR, editors. Pediatric prevention of atherosclerotic cardiovascular disease. New York: Oxford University Press Inc; 2008.

36. Jokela M, Kivimäki M, Elovainio M, et al. Body mass index in adolescence and number of children in adulthood. Epidemiology 2007;18(5):599–606.

37. Unger RH. Reinventing type 2 diabetes: pathogenesis, treatment, and prevention. JAMA 2008;299:1185–7.

38. Nguyen QM, Srinivasan SR, Xu JH, et al. Influence of childhood parental history of type 2 diabetes on the pre-diabetic and diabetic status in adulthood: the Bogalusa Heart Study. Eur J Epidemiol 2009;24:537–9.

39. Nguyen QM, Srinivasan SR, Xu JH, et al. Fasting plasma glucose levels within the normoglycemic range in childhood as a predictor of pre-diabetes and type 2 diabetes in adulthood: the Bogalusa Heart Study. Arch Pediatr Adolesc Med 2010; 164:124–8.

40. Nguyen QM, Srinivasan SR, Xu JH, et al. Utility of childhood glucose homeostasis variables in predicting adult diabetes and related cardiometabolic risk factors: the Bogalusa Heart Study. Diabetes Care 2010;33:670–5.

41. Nguyen QM, Srinivasan SR, Xu JH, et al. Changes in risk variables of metabolic syndrome since childhood in pre-diabetic and type 2 diabetic subjects: the Bogalusa Heart Study. Diabetes Care 2008;31:2044–9.

42. Twigg SM, Kamp MC, Davis TM, et al, Australian Diabetes Society, Australian Diabetes Educators Association. Prediabetes: a position statement from the Australian Diabetes Society and Australian Diabetes Educators Association. Med J Aust 2007;186:461–5.

43. Chen W, Srinivasan SR, Elkasabany A, et al. Cardiovascular risk factors clustering features of insulin resistance syndrome (Syndrome X) in a biracial (Black-White) population of children, adolescents, and young adults: the Bogalusa Heart Study. Am J Epidemiol 1999;150:667–74.

44. DECODE Study Group, the European Diabetes Epidemiology Group. Glucose tolerance and cardiovascular mortality: comparison of fasting and 2-hour diagnostic criteria. Arch Intern Med 2001;161:397–405.

45. American Diabetes Association. Diagnosis and classification of diabetes mellitus. Diabetes Care 2010;33(Suppl 1):S62–9.

46. Gillman MW. Predicting pre-diabetes and diabetes: can we do it? Is it worth it? Arch Pediatr Adolesc Med 2010;164:198–9.

47. Downey AM, Frank GC, Webber LS, et al. Implementation of "Heart Smart:" a cardiovascular school health promotion program. J Sch Health 1987;57: 98–104.

48. Berenson GS. Cardiovascular health promotion for children: a model for a Parish (County)-wide program (implementation and preliminary results). Prev Cardiol 2010;13:23–8.

Index

Note: Page numbers of article titles are in **boldface** type.

Integrated
diabetes
coverage
from Elsevier

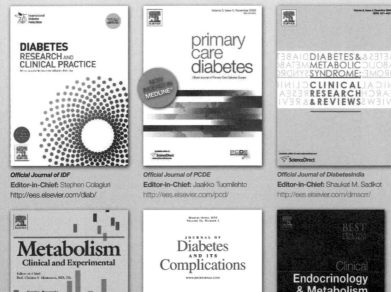

Official Journal of IDF
Editor-in-Chief: Stephen Colagiuri
http://ees.elsevier.com/diab/

Official Journal of PCDE
Editor-in-Chief: Jaakko Tuomilehto
http://ees.elsevier.com/pcd/

Official Journal of DiabetesIndia
Editor-in-Chief: Shaukat M. Sadikot
http://ees.elsevier.com/dmscrr/

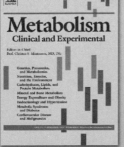

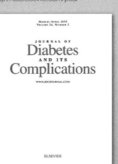

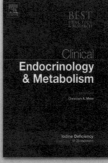

Editor-in-Chief: Christos S. Mantzoros
http://ees.elsevier.com/metabolism/

Editor-in-Chief: Philip Raskin
http://ees.elsevier.com/jdc/

Editor-in-Chief: Christoph A. Meier
www.elsevier.com/locate/beem/

Moving?

Make sure your subscription moves with you!

To notify us of your new address, find your **Clinics Account Number** (located on your mailing label above your name), and contact customer service at:

Email: journalscustomerservice-usa@elsevier.com

800-654-2452 (subscribers in the U.S. & Canada)
314-447-8871 (subscribers outside of the U.S. & Canada)

Fax number: 314-447-8029

Elsevier Health Sciences Division
Subscription Customer Service
3251 Riverport Lane
Maryland Heights, MO 63043

*To ensure uninterrupted delivery of your subscription, please notify us at least 4 weeks in advance of move.